PRAISE FOR

The Mommy Diet

"As a mom of four, I know how important exercise and diet are during all phases of pregnancy. Going to the doctor is crucial but sometimes there are those moments where you just want to hang with other moms who've been there and who have the benefit of experience and plain common sense to talk to. Alison Sweeney's *The Mommy Diet* is like having that best friend right there anytime you are looking for advice and mom tips. There's nothing Hollywood about this Hollywood mom; she's the real thing, and I for one would've loved to have had her book when I had my kids!"

—Marlee Matlin, Academy Award–winning
actress and author of *I'll Scream Later*

"*The Mommy Diet* is the next 'must-have' pregnancy guide/ new mommy bible! Ali has perfectly captured the information mommies-to-be and new mommies need to know and her soothing voice and demeanor really shine through at a highly sensitive time when we need to hear it the most."

—Holly Robinson Peete, actress, author,
philanthropist, co-host of *The Talk*,
mom of 4

The
Mommy Diet

A month-by-month plan
for a healthy body and mind
before, during, *and* after pregnancy

Alison Sweeney
with Christie Matheson

G

Gallery Books
New York London Toronto Sydney

Gallery Books
A Division of Simon and Schuster, Inc.
1230 Avenue of the Americas
New York, NY 10020

First Gallery Books hardcover edition January 2011

GALLERY BOOKS and colophon are registered trademarks of
Simon & Schuster, Inc.

For information about special discounts for bulk purchases,
please contact Simon & Schuster Special Sales at 1-866-506-1949 or
business@simonandschuster.com.

The Simon & Schuster Speakers Bureau can bring authors to your
live event. For more information or to book an event contact the
Simon & Schuster Speakers Bureau at 1-866-248-3049 or
visit our website at www.simonspeakers.com.

Designed by Jaime Putorti
Illustrations by Amy Saidens

Manufactured in the United States of America

10   9   8   7   6   5   4   3   2   1

Library of Congress Cataloging-in-Publication Data

Sweeney, Alison
The mommy diet / Alison Sweeney.
p. cm.
Pregnancy—Nutritional aspects—Popular works. 2. Pregnant women—Health and hygiene—Popular works. I. Title.
RG559.S94 2010
618.2'42—dc22   2010015908

ISBN: 978-1-4391-8094-5
ISBN: 978-1-4391-8095-2 (ebook)

Contents

To Ben and Megan,
who inspire me every day
to be the best mom I can be

Introduction

Having a baby is a life-changing experience like no other. I'll never forget the night my first baby—my son, Ben, who is now five—was born, and the moment when the nurse brought him to my room, handed him to me, and left me alone with him. As she walked away and closed the door, all I could think was, *Where are you going, lady? Who's going to make sure I don't harm this innocent child? I am not qualified to be in charge here!* A baby completely rocks your world. Mostly in a wonderful, amazing way.

Let's be honest, though. Being pregnant and taking care of your beautiful little baby also mean some serious changes to your body, your sleep schedule, and your ability to take care of yourself. That's normal, of course. Don't feel like you're alone in this, or like you're the only mom who can't figure it all out and get it together right away. *Everyone* goes through this stage, and that's what this book is all about: You can still look and feel great! I'm not going to tell you it's supereasy to eat perfectly, or that you'll get your body back in two weeks, or that you'll find countless opportunities for exercise and pampering every day. And no, you're not always going to look like a perfect catalog mom, strolling casually down Rodeo Drive with a beautifully dressed, napping child in a fancy stroller.

The brutal truth is that your hair and makeup won't be flawless, your socks sometimes won't match, it takes many months to get in shape, and you'll often be wondering when and where you can get another snack. (Especially if you're breastfeeding . . . you'll be thinking about snacks a lot!)

Now I'll give you the good news: You *can* eat healthfully, be physically fit, look great, and find time to take care of *you* while at the same time learning to be a terrific new mom. Once you enter the incredible world of motherhood, your priorities shift, as well they should. But you can't leave *you* out of the equation. This is not at all selfish! Believe me, you *and* your family will be so much happier if you give yourself the attention you deserve and find ways to look and feel fabulous. I want to help you do that.

If this is your first pregnancy (congratulations!), you're going to be reading a lot of books and getting tons of advice along the way. I read anything and everything I could get my hands on during my first pregnancy. And I got plenty of great advice—but I also got advice from many of the overly excited, usually well-meaning people who feel compelled to preach to every pregnant woman they see that she *must* do this and must *never* do that. You'll hear people issue proclamations about everything from whether you can have a cup of coffee in the morning to the pros and cons of immunizations. I'm sure you've already run into this type. Well, that's not how I roll. And that's not the kind of advice I give. Consider this book a safe space: I am not here to issue mandates or make you feel guilty or scared or confused. I definitely have opinions about all the main maternity issues, but I managed to survive two pregnancies mostly by going with my gut. I encourage you to do the same thing.

So what is *The Mommy Diet*? It's not just a weight-loss book, though it is packed with information about how to eat right and get in shape. It's about a "diet" of nutrition, fitness, and self-care that women can follow in order to look and feel fantastic—before and during pregnancy, and after giving birth. The focus of *The Mommy Diet* is getting you physically and mentally healthy and keeping you that way. It's not about making you instantly skinny—sorry, that's just not possible or healthy—though it will help you slim down for sure, in a positive, attainable way.

With targeted advice and proven strategies for every stage along the way, *The Mommy Diet* will guide you through the three trimesters of pregnancy, the early postpregnancy recovery period, and the first nine months of being a mommy. Just as gestation takes nine months, it might take another nine months to feel "normal" (or better!) again—though you'll be feeling really, really good much sooner than that if you follow the wellness plan outlined in these pages. *The Mommy Diet* will help you to be fit and healthy during pregnancy, lose weight sensibly after the baby comes, and look and feel great with tips for fashion, beauty, and self-care throughout the process.

There's also a chapter for moms who are more than nine months postpartum and think they've held on to their baby weight for too long—this more intense "kick-start" program can help any mom get herself into shape and start feeling better. And once you've attained your goals and just want to stay healthy, fit, and happy as the journey of motherhood continues, there's a chapter about that, too.

The tips in *The Mommy Diet* are realistic, affordable, and doable for any mom. It's an easy—and inexpensive—"diet" to follow. Because even though we'd all love to have endless time and money to devote to looking and feeling great, very few real moms and moms-to-be do.

I certainly know what it's like to be busy. I'm a working mom with two kids (Ben, five, and Megan, one) and two jobs (I'm the host of the NBC show *The Biggest Loser* and I play Sami Brady on *Days of our Lives*). I get what you're going through! When it comes to parenting, I am in the trenches—dealing with middle-of-the-night feedings and diaper changes and spit-ups, just trying to get a little sleep. And like most moms, soon after my kids were born I did start wondering . . . When will I get my figure back? *How* do I get my figure back? When do I have *time* to get my figure back? Will I ever have a chance to get a manicure again? And what the hell did this baby do to my stomach muscles? Unfortunately, I didn't have a magic button I could press to get back into shape magically fast. (I wish!)

Even though I am just another working mom in many ways, I'm lucky to have access to Hollywood's best trainers and nutritionists (there are perks to starring in a hit weight-loss reality show!), as well as hair and makeup artists, stylists, and other experts who have given me tons of great advice, tips, and tricks for getting and staying in shape and taking care of myself. I've also learned so much from being part of *The Biggest Loser*. I've totally reevaluated my approach to diet and nutrition—in fact, I ate so much better during my second pregnancy (and got my body back much faster than I did with my first pregnancy) thanks in part to the knowledge I've gained from the experts on the show. So I want to share all that—plus helpful hints from my own experiences, and other real moms' experiences—with you. After all, we moms need to stick together and help one another out. Moms should never have to go it alone.

The Mommy Diet is organized in five sections: before pregnancy, during pregnancy, the nine months after pregnancy, a kick-start program for anytime, and a maintenance program for all moms. The pregnancy section is divided into three chapters (for the first, second, and third trimesters), and the post-pregnancy section has month-by-month chapters, because things change quite a bit during that time.

In each chapter, I cover fitness and food, with specific plans for working out and eating, as well as general tips. I also cover fashion (because you want to look good throughout this process, and you can!), self-care (all the little things you can do to pamper yourself, plus take care of your skin, hair, and nails—which isn't frivolous but truly necessary if you want to maintain a positive outlook), and romance (another key to feeling great while you're pregnant and as a new mom).

You can read the whole thing at once and then go back to the different sections as needed, or just take a few minutes to read whichever section applies to you at the moment. When you're a new mom, you often have only a minute or two at a time to read, so just flip to the chapter for whatever phase you're in and get tips to help you right now. And you can always check in at alisonsweeney.com for more recipes, more exercise ideas (some moves are better explained in video than print!), and an online community of moms who are also following *The Mommy Diet*. It's a good place to go for up-to-the-minute food and fitness news, feedback to your personal questions, connections with moms in your area, and great support whenever you need it.

Before you begin, though, you need to understand the bottom line when it comes to taking good care of yourself: You have to want to do this, and you have to acknowledge that you're the only one who can do it. You're the one who will have to get to the gym or a yoga class, or get out for a walk or a run. You're the one who will have to buy the healthier groceries—and eat them (not junk!), too. You're the one who will have to make sure you're getting *you* time. No one can do it for you.

I remember being on set at *Days of Our Lives* a year after Ben was born. At that time I was not feeling confident about my figure—and the "I just had a baby" excuse was starting to wear thin. I was in a scene with a gorgeous, fit actress, and as she left the studio, I saw all the cast and crew members watching her walk away. She was a head-turner, for sure. I said out loud what all the women watching her were probably thinking: "I would do anything to have that body." And then, after a beat, realizing that everyone had heard me, I joked, ". . . except eat right and work out." It got the whole crew laughing, and then we went back to work.

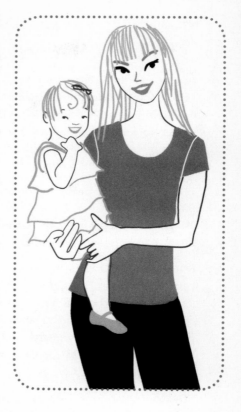

I thought about that incident a lot that night. It was a really big awakening for me. I realized that I *can* look like that, if I'm willing to do what it takes to get there. And so can you. You *can* go after what you want. It's not about secret Hollywood grapefruit diets, buying tapeworms on the Internet, or selling your soul to the devil. It simply comes down to making the decision to fight for what you want. Whatever motivates you, whether it's fitting into those size twenty-seven jeans again (or for the first time), or being able to chase your child around the playground without getting exhausted, you have to decide what your goals are and find the will to go for them. With the help of this book, you have all the tools you need to get there.

MOMMY DIET EXPERTS

As I mentioned earlier, I was able to reach my goals with the help of some amazing experts who gave me guidance on fitness, nutrition, style, and more. I'm lucky to know them—and in this book much of the advice I share comes from them. Here's the scoop on the incredible people who contributed wisdom to *The Mommy Diet*.

JESSE BRUNE is a trainer, nutrition expert, and Le Cordon Bleu–trained chef. He starred in Bravo Television's hit series *Workout*, and he has been featured on *The Bonnie Hunt Show*, *Access Hollywood*, and E!'s *Red Carpet Oscar Special*.

ROCCO DISPIRITO is an award-winning chef and bestselling cookbook author. He starred in the reality television series *The Restaurant*, he was a contestant on *Dancing with the Stars*, and he has appeared many times on *Top Chef* and *The Biggest Loser*, which is where I got to know him. His latest book is *Now Eat This! 150 of America's Favorite Comfort Foods, All Under 350 Calories*.

CORINA DURAN, my makeup artist, has been doing my makeup since I started on *Days of our Lives* in 1993. She has done makeup for movies such as *Hitch*, *Serena*, *I Now Pronounce You Chuck & Larry*, and *Paul Blart: Mall Cop*, and for the television show *King of Queens*.

ELISE GULAN is a trainer and the creator of the DVDs *Element: Ballet Conditioning*, *Ultimate Body: Yoga Fitness*, and *SHAPE: 20-Minute Makeover*. She has been featured as a health and fitness expert on *ABC News*, *E! News*, *EXTRA*, and *CBS News*, and in *Allure*, *Elle*, *Glamour*, *Self*, *Shape*, *Women's Health*, and *People*.

→

MEG WERNER MORETA is a registered dietitian with a master's degree in human nutrition. She currently has a private practice in Beverly Hills, and she has practiced at Cedars-Sinai and USC. She works frequently with Dr. Rob Huizenga from *The Biggest Loser*, and she was the nutritionist for *Dance Your Ass Off* on the Oxygen Network.

STEVIE SANT'ANGELO, my trainer, recently gained widespread attention for helping Jennifer Love Hewitt slim down. I met her through *The Biggest Loser* trainer Jillian Michaels.

LIZA WHITCRAFT is my stylist for *The Biggest Loser*. She has also dressed Elle Macpherson and Kobe Bryant and styled for commercials, photo shoots, television, and movies. And George Clooney directed her as she played herself—a wardrobe stylist—in the HBO series *Unscripted*.

Before Pregnancy

Deciding you want to get pregnant—or thinking it might be a possibility soon—is a big milestone. Get ready for your life to change! And until then, enjoy being master of your own body and your own schedule, because that won't last forever. In the meantime, you need to start taking very good care of yourself—well *before* you're actually knocked up. There are many reasons to do this.

First, you want your baby to have the healthiest possible environment in which to grow from the moment of conception. This means getting your body ready now!

Second, chances are you don't know exactly when you'll get pregnant. Sure, it could take a while, but it could also happen right away. You never know, so be prepared. If your pregnancy comes as a surprise, please don't worry. Plenty of healthy babies are born every day to parents who nine months earlier had no idea they were conceiving a child. Still, you want to give your child every advantage you can, right? So we'll focus on helping you be the healthiest host you can be for the little person who will soon be spending the better part of a year inside of you.

Third, your chances of getting pregnant and having a complication-free pregnancy are greatest if you are healthy and fit. Of course, being healthy and fit doesn't mean you'll get pregnant instantly, but it does help. The first time I tried to get pregnant, it took about a year, and I remember being frustrated when my friends got pregnant more quickly, while I kept seeing one line in the window of the pregnancy test instead of two. If you're in the same situation, it's best to get past the frustration and to focus on your own journey. Don't compare your path to anyone else's. (I know that's not the easiest advice to take, but I'm going to offer it anyway.) Since I couldn't make my body get pregnant, I had to focus on the other things I could control, like my health, fitness, and nutrition. I reduced my alcohol intake, too, by mostly cutting out my glass of wine with dinner and skipping the cocktails when I was out with friends. Not to be a downer, but if you have any other unhealthy habits, like smoking or taking drugs of any kind, I highly suggest you deal with them now, before you are pregnant, so your body will be healthier and so you don't have to deal with the stress of withdrawal on top of everything else.

Fourth, being healthy before you get pregnant makes it way easier to stay active and fit during pregnancy, which, in turn, means you'll get your body back a whole lot faster after the baby is born. (I know that seems like a long way off right now, but trust me: You want things to be as easy as possible once your bundle of joy arrives!)

I could list about a hundred more reasons, but the point is that everything you do now really matters. And a recent study (published in 2009 in the *British Medical Journal*) found that most women don't follow the lifestyle and health guidelines suggested for women who are trying to conceive. Oops. Let's work on changing that. I want you to have the best and healthiest pregnancy possible, so here are tips to help you set yourself up for that.

Fitness

I'm excited for you—seriously—because if you're reading this before you get pregnant, you have an amazing opportunity right now to start, amp up, or focus on your fitness routine. As a busy mom, I admit that I sometimes miss those times before I had kids when I could work out (or do anything) pretty much whenever I wanted. If I felt like hitting a certain spin or yoga class, or I suddenly had the urge to spend a few hours at the gym or go for a jog, no problem. Knowing what I know now, I wish I'd spent a little more time working out back then, when there was no need to worry about who else needed me. I could just leave my husband a message (this was before texting—remember that?) and do it! Of course, I wouldn't trade my current situation for anything, but I want you to enjoy this freedom, and use it to concentrate on yourself. The more active and fit you are before you're pregnant, the more you can keep doing while you're pregnant—which, again, is so good for you and your baby. Here are a few things to think about.

1. Keep up—or start—a regular cardio habit. Pregnancy and childbirth are often compared to running a marathon, and you wouldn't try to run a marathon without training, would you? (If you did, it would hurt. A lot.)

One of the best ways to get ready for your endurance event is with regular cardiovascular exercise (think walking, hiking, spinning, running, elliptical, stair climber, cross-country skiing). Do it at least three times per week for thirty minutes. Preferably more like five times (or more) per week. Not only is it good for you, but it will make you feel fantastic.

If you've never worked out before, start slowly and build up your cardio regimen. If you're working out once or twice a week now, hey, let's step it up a bit. There's no downside. And if you already have a great fitness routine, don't stop!

2. Keep up—or add—regular strength training. This doesn't mean you have to lift heavy weights and bulk up. Not even close. I'm talking about things like Pilates, yoga, Bar Method, Core Fusion, circuit training with light weights, and abs classes . . . anything that focuses on strengthening your muscles. Yoga, by the way, is one of the best things you can start doing now. It helps you get strong, and it also helps you learn how to breathe slowly and calmly through anything, which will come in handy down the road when you're having an intense contraction.

3. Always remember how important exercise is, especially now. It may seem unnecessary. You're about to gain thirty pounds, so why bother working out? But it is *not* a waste of

time. I promise you'll be grateful to be as fit as you can be going into one of the most physically strenuous times of your life.

4. This isn't exactly an exercise tip, but it is most definitely related to your overall fitness and health: If you happen to be a smoker, please, please, *please* stop smoking now. Get that out of the way before you're pregnant. Do it. This is not negotiable. Okay, I promised not to issue mandates, but I am going to break that promise just for one second right here. Do not smoke if you are pregnant. Please. Okay, that's it. I'm done.

Food

I wish I could tell you to go crazy and enjoy all the foods (and drinks!) you have to skip during pregnancy. Sorry, I can't do that. When you're trying to get pregnant, you need to start eating like you're already pregnant—because you may not realize you're pregnant until you're many weeks along. Besides, this is not a time when you want to be eating and drinking to excess and setting yourself up for possible unhealthy weight gain. Which brings us to the following food for thought.

1. Because dieting to lose weight while pregnant is a no-no, and because it's easier to get pregnant and have a complication-free pregnancy if you are at a healthy weight, now is the time to focus on reaching your healthy weight, if you're not there already. If you are underweight, this means gaining a few pounds,

and if you are overweight, it's a good opportunity to lose a few pounds. See your doctor, tell her you're thinking about getting pregnant, and have an honest conversation about your weight and whether you need to change your eating habits. Remember, it's what you eat that has the biggest impact on weight gain or weight loss. If you're already at a healthy weight, that's great! This is the perfect time to make sure you're eating the healthy, nutritious foods that are best for you.

2. Get 400 micrograms of folate or folic acid per day. You may have heard that folic acid is a key nutrient to take in while you're pregnant, because it helps to prevent neural tube defects (serious birth defects). Well, you really should be getting

MD EATS: ✳ *Simple Folate-Filled Salad*

Serves 1 or 2

This salad is easy to make, and a good way to get lots of nutrients—including a dose of extra folate—into your system.

> 2 cups raw spinach leaves (100 micrograms folate)
> 2 tablespoons orange juice (10 micrograms folate)
> 1 teaspoon olive oil
> Salt and pepper to taste
> 1 cup whole strawberries, hulled and chopped
>   (36 micrograms folate)

Toss the spinach leaves with the juice, oil, salt, and pepper so the leaves are all lightly coated. Add the strawberries, toss gently, and serve.

MD EXTRA: ❋ *Banish the Bread Basket*

From here on out, let's make a deal never to eat the bread they give you at restaurants. It's almost always completely worthless calories. My husband calls it filler. Save your appetite for the yummy thing you're about to order. Don't waste your appetite on those empty carbs.

that daily dose of folic acid well before you're pregnant, because the baby's neural tube forms very early in pregnancy. You can get it from foods—leafy green veggies (such as spinach), citrus fruits, beans, strawberries, and enriched cereals—but because it's tough to get the recommended daily amount just from food, most doctors suggest taking a folic acid supplement or a multivitamin with folic acid. Talk to your doc to see what she suggests for you.

3. Make your carbs whole grains. This is one of the simplest changes to make if you want a healthier diet, and it's a great habit to adopt now and keep forever. Instead of white bread, regular pasta, and white rice, have whole wheat bread, whole wheat pasta, and brown rice. You'll get more fiber and nutrients and fewer empty calories.

4. I'll say this again: Eat lots of veggies and fruits. Get in the habit of eating at least three servings of vegetables and two servings of fruit per day. If you're not doing this now (really pay attention to quantity—you might think you're doing it, but you

MD EATS: ☀ *Sanov Family Oatmeal Pancakes*

Serves 6

This recipe has been a favorite in my husband's family since the 1970s. When my in-laws first made it for me, I was blown away. They're so light and delicious, and they are a good source of whole grains. Don't be alarmed if the batter seems runny and lumpy. That's because of the oatmeal, and that's exactly what it should be like. If you make sure the griddle or pan is hot enough, each quarter cup of batter will make two silver-dollar-sized pancakes. I like to eat two of these with a drizzle of maple syrup, fruit salad, and yogurt for a satisfying breakfast. (I don't suggest a huge stack of them—think of them as a breakfast side dish, not the main course.) Take the time for a leisurely (and healthy) morning treat now!

> *2 cups cooled cooked oatmeal (cook according to*
> *the directions on the oatmeal box)*
> *1½ cups milk*
> *3/8 cup safflower or vegetable oil*
> *2 eggs*
> *1/3 cup whole wheat flour*
> *2 tablespoons powdered milk*
> *¼ teaspoon salt*

In a medium bowl, mix the cooled cooked oatmeal with the milk. Whisk in the oil. In a separate small bowl, beat the eggs. Make sure the oatmeal is cool (or it will cook the eggs) and stir the beaten eggs into the oatmeal mixture. Stir in the whole wheat flour, the powdered milk, and the salt.

Heat a griddle or skillet on medium-high heat, and spray lightly with cooking spray or oil. When the griddle or pan is hot, use about ¼ cup of batter to make two pancakes, and cook for 1 to 2 minutes on each side, until golden brown. Stir the batter occasionally as it sits while you're making the first batches of pancakes.

may not be), make yourself do it for a few weeks until it becomes automatic. Start with breakfast—it's easy to have berries or a banana with yogurt or cereal. At lunch, think about salads and veggie-filled soups. For dinner, always make vegetables and salads part of the plan. Snack on fruits and veggies, too! Whenever you're making a salad, don't use iceberg or romaine, because they offer no nutritional value. Use butter (or Boston) lettuce, arugula, or mixed greens that give you some health bang for your buck. Mix in some raw spinach leaves, too.

MD EATS: ✳ *When to Opt for Organic*

Organic foods are getting easier to find, so I encourage you to choose organic (which means free of chemical pesticides and fertilizers) over conventional whenever you can in order to keep unhealthy chemicals out of your body. Here are the fruits and veggies Meg Moreta says tend to be most contaminated—so if you're deciding which organic foods to prioritize, these are the most important.

FRUITS	VEGETABLES
Apples	Celery
Pears	Lettuce
Grapes	Potatoes
Peaches	Sweet bell peppers
Nectarines	
Strawberries	
Cherries	
Tomatoes (technically a fruit, not a veggie!)	

5. Say adios to your wine. Ouch. This could be a tough one for those of us who enjoy a few glasses of wine, or cocktails, or whatever. But seriously, you may be many weeks into your pregnancy before you realize you're pregnant, and getting tipsy just isn't a good idea near the start of pregnancy (or anytime during pregnancy, for that matter). I would occasionally have one glass of wine with dinner while I was trying to get pregnant, but for anything more than that, the risk just didn't seem worth it to me. This is another topic to discuss with your doctor, please. The good news: If you don't drink, you never have to worry about a hangover. . . .

6. Consider starting a calcium supplement and a prenatal vitamin. For calcium, my doctor recommended those chocolate Viactiv Calcium Soft Chews. They taste pretty good! As for prenatal vitamins, the general recommendation is to start taking them at least three months before conception, so your body has all the nutrients you need for those crucial first few weeks and months of baby development. Some doctors believe morning sickness can be partially attributed to your body getting used to prenatal vitamins, so go ahead and start them before you're actually pregnant and give your body a chance to get used to them before all the other craziness begins. Talk to your doctor about what makes sense for you.

Fashion

You've been dressing yourself for a long time and your body hasn't started changing due to pregnancy yet, so do you really need *Mommy Diet* fashion advice now? Well, maybe. Fashion is pretty important. Like it or not, what you wear speaks volumes about who you are. When you get pregnant, and then after you have a baby, it's not always easy to pull together a great look, especially if you're not already confident about what works for you. Take this opportunity—when you're not yet carrying around extra pounds and you don't have a crying baby demanding your attention—to get your style together.

1. Know how to dress to impress. Yes, I'm a big fan of comfort clothes. (I wear four-inch heels at work with my tall costars, but I wear my Chuck Taylors or flip-flops almost every day at home.) But when you're going out on the town, practice putting a little effort into how you come across. When you're dealing with a weeks-old baby, you might not have it in you to pull together a whole ensemble . . . so while you don't have any excuses, come on, step it up a notch!

2. Clean out your closet. Make room for maternity clothes, and get rid of all the stuff you'll never wear again. You know there are pieces hanging around in there that should *never* see the light of day. Why are you clinging to them? I'll suggest doing a more thorough closet "edit" later, but for now, just try to clean out the crap. Give it away or donate it. Rip it off like a Band-Aid! Invite a friend over to help you with the tough de-

cisions, and maybe have one of those very few glasses of wine you're allowed right now to make the good-byes a little easier.

3. Don't go on any shopping sprees right now. Your body is going to change soon, so why spend a lot of money on pieces you won't be able to wear for the next year? You might not like them anymore when they do fit again. Go through your closet (post clean-out), try things on, and figure out what style resonates best with you. Do you gravitate to cashmere sweaters and pearls? Or funky T-shirts? Or girly dresses? Or tailored pieces? This is the time to recognize and *own* your style. Then when you're shopping for maternity clothes, keep that fashion sense in mind.

Self-Care

You'll soon understand that having plenty of time to take care of yourself is a luxury, so take advantage of it while you can.

1. Do whatever relaxes you. And do it often. Maybe it's going to yoga, maybe it's watching a silly movie, maybe it's going to bed early with a great book. Studies show the less stressed you are, the easier time you'll have getting pregnant. This is a good habit to get into, because avoiding stress during pregnancy is good for you and your baby. Think about it for a minute or two: What *really* puts you into your most mellow, chilled-out, happy mood?

2. Clear your home of toxic chemicals. Yikes, what toxic chemicals? Unfortunately, most of us are living with a lot of them. Believe it or not, the indoor air in homes is generally two to five times more polluted than outdoor air. So just be aware of what you're bringing into your home. Choose natural and organic cleaning products. If you're painting a room, use *only* low-VOC paints (VOC stands for volatile organic compound; VOCs can cause everything from headaches and nausea to liver and kidney damage). Stay away from chemical air fresheners, and if you get your clothes dry-cleaned, go to a "green" dry cleaner that doesn't use the chemical perchloroethylene (just ask them if they use "perc"—if they say they don't know or tell you it's harmless, go to a different cleaner).

3. If you wear acrylic nails, now is the time to get rid of them. It's really not good to breathe in those fumes while you're pregnant, so you might as well get started on giving your nails a chance to grow back on their own. If you like polish on your nails, pick out shades you like from brands that are free of formaldehyde, toluene, and dibutyl phthlate (aka DBP).

4. Go to bed earlier. A healthy lifestyle includes plenty of sleep, and I know I didn't always get enough sleep before I had children. (I still don't always get enough sleep, but for different reasons.) Sleeping well means getting sick less often and having way more energy; both are very important as you begin this new adventure. Plus, staying out really late doesn't work well when you're pregnant or a new mom, so the early-to-bed habit is a good one to start now.

5. If you're having a hard time getting pregnant, or if you need help getting pregnant, take it easy on yourself. It can be an emotional and hormonal roller coaster well above and beyond the hormonal ups and downs of pregnancy. If you have a miscarriage while trying to get pregnant, give yourself time to grieve and heal—but also realize that it's very common (it happens in 15 to 20 percent of recognized pregnancies, and more like 50 percent of all pregnancies), and that you can and likely will go on to have a wonderful and healthy pregnancy.

This can be such a tough road, and I applaud your strength as you continue on it. As you do, unless your doctor specifically tells you that you need to back off your workout routine (and I highly recommend including her in your decisions at this point), you can use workouts to help you burn your stress, tension, and sadness.

Eating healthfully can also help you feel better about yourself. I'm not going to lie: Chocolate does have some emotionally healing properties and health benefits. But only when you consume it within reasonable limits. A little makes you feel better, but if you go beyond just a bit, the more you eat, the worse you'll feel. (Remember that just 1 ounce of chocolate has about 150 calories.) So enjoy a bite or two if it's your favorite and you're having a crappy day. I love the dark chocolate from Trader Joe's. (Dark chocolate contains antioxidants that are good for you.) I have a bar of it in my dressing room at *Days,* and I break off a little piece when I need a taste of something sweet. One bar lasts a long time. But if there's something you can't resist (for me it's Red Velvet *anything!*) and you are likely to polish off a huge chocolate bar or pint of ice cream in one sitting when you're feeling down, keep it out of the house.

Romance

In theory, this should be a very romantic time for you and your partner. You're planning for the future and thinking about the amazing family you will create together. Plus, you're having lots of sex! Woohoo! Everything is perfect!

Please don't be disappointed if this isn't the scenario you're experiencing. Unfortunately, it's not totally realistic. Along with all the planning comes a fair amount of stress, whether you're worried about money or time or difficulty conceiving. And all that sex? Well, it's nice, but it can also start to feel like a chore if you let it. (Somehow, "Honey, we need to do it *now* because I'm ovulating" isn't as much of a turn-on as more spontaneous forms of foreplay.)

Before this all becomes a major bummer, try to remember everything that is romantic about trying to have a baby. Focus on the positive, and use this time to ignite passion in the bedroom. A healthy sex life is an important part of any relationship, so have fun; here are a few tips to help you and your partner enjoy the process.

1. Remember that you're in this together. Yes, you'll be doing most of the work for the next nine months. Still, you're deciding to start a family together and that's an incredible thing. Talk about it, share anything that's stressing you out, and be

there to support each other. If you're frustrated with anything (like it's taking longer than you want to conceive), try not to take it out on your partner. Remain allies and best friends!

2. Don't let sex become too clinical. Even if you're sticking to a schedule, keep the romance alive! Light some candles, have a date first, play sexy games, and most important, focus on being with your partner—not just the intended outcome.

3. Spend time focusing on yourselves and your marriage before you try to have kids. This was really important to my husband, and I'm so glad he encouraged us to think about it. We worked on our careers and took time to travel and felt like we were really *ready* to focus on a new family member before we tried to conceive.

You have to approach family life in whatever way works for you, but Dave and I are both so glad we did things the way we did—not rushing to have kids, and getting to do things that we wanted to do. It may be another ten years before we are able to go back to Europe, and next time we'll probably go with our kids, but until then I have wonderful memories of seeing amazing Parisian architecture and enjoying those fabulous dinners in Italy (during which I probably violated every rule in this book, but that's what Italy is for, right?). Whatever it is that you want to do that isn't quite as easy or practical when you have a baby . . . do it *now*! Have some adventures together, take lots of photos, and know that you'll always be glad you did.

Pregnancy

First Trimester

Congratulations! You are beginning a huge adventure. It's thrilling to find out that you're pregnant. Of course, it can also be overwhelming and scary. And the changes that you know are coming to your body—not to mention the fatigue and morning sickness I'm sure you've heard you might experience—are daunting! But if that ever starts to freak you out, just focus on this amazing thing that your body is doing. You're growing another person. Wow.

Maybe you've been trying to get pregnant for a while, or maybe it was a surprise. It took me almost a year to get pregnant the first time, and when I finally saw that little pink line on the pregnancy test I was beyond ecstatic. I couldn't wait to tell my husband, Dave. Truly, I couldn't wait. He picked me up to go to a basketball game and I *wanted* to wait and tell him when we were face-to-face, not while he was driving, but I was bursting with the news. I held it in just long enough for us to get on the freeway and then I couldn't hold it in anymore—but at that point he couldn't even pull over. He was overjoyed, but also frustrated because he had to keep his eyes on the road, so he couldn't hug me or even look me in the eye to celebrate the moment.

It's so exciting. But let me warn you, if you haven't realized it already: The early stages of pregnancy can be physically and emotionally exhausting. When I first found out I was pregnant, I tried desperately to notice changes in my body immediately. For a few weeks, I wondered if the test result was even accurate because I didn't feel any different. And then . . . wham. Dave and I came home from a date night and Dave realized that our DVR hadn't recorded my favorite show, *The Amazing Race*. Minor bummer, right? Well, I literally started to weep, soap opera style. Tears were streaming down my face; my body was shaking. I cried uncontrollably for more than an hour. I know, I know. Crazy. (Dave was trying to console me while turning his face away to hide his laughter.) By the end of my little bout of hysteria, I was laughing at myself, although still crying a little at the same time. And that was my rude awakening to the wild hormonal changes my body was experiencing.

That happened when I was ten weeks along, and I hadn't told anyone at work yet that I was pregnant. I woke up the next morning, after my crying jag, looked in the mirror, and almost freaked out again. I didn't even recognize my own face. I was a disaster! Not only were my eyes puffy and bloodshot, I had about a million burst capillaries in the delicate skin underneath them. I looked like a train wreck. It was horrifying. (Okay, it probably wasn't as bad as I thought it was, but— hello—my hormones had kicked in, so it seemed like the end of the world to me.)

When I went to work at *Days*, I had to offer some sort of explanation. I could hardly just say, "Oh, I sobbed for an hour last night because TiVo didn't tape my show." That would have sounded insane. I wasn't ready to reveal that I was pregnant—I am superstitious about stuff like that. I wanted to wait until the end of the first trimester before telling anyone, which is pretty standard. Your doctor will explain that you just never know what's going to happen and that the first trimester is the most unpredictable. Anyway, even though I was only two weeks away from the big revelation, I still tried to play it off while on set the next day. I admitted that I'd been crying but didn't really explain why. Then I spent all day paranoid (notice a trend here?) that my coworkers would come up with their own reasons for why I was crying, like I was having marital problems or something. So I held out for about three more days and then announced my pregnancy, and explained why I was really crying. It definitely cracks people up to hear how devastated I was to miss my favorite show. That's how I learned a very important lesson: Those hysterical incidents are easier to deal with if you can laugh at yourself afterward.

Fitness

Talk to your doctor about exercise as soon as you find out that you're pregnant, and keep talking to her about it throughout your pregnancy. For most women, exercising while pregnant is fine—great, in fact—but we're all different, and you need to make sure you're doing it safely and heeding the specific precautions that apply to you.

So, assuming you get the okay from your doc, if you thought pregnancy was going to be a nine-month break from all physical activity . . . nope! Soldiers don't take naps before going into battle, and let me tell you, this is a battle. For a superhealthy pregnancy—and for a much, much, *much* easier time getting back in shape after pregnancy—regular exercise is key.

If you had a good workout routine going before you got pregnant, you can keep up with most of your activities (see MD Moves, page 21, for some important modifications). And if you didn't work out at all before pregnancy, there's no time like the present to focus on getting healthy and easing into a gentle workout plan!

However, whether you were active before or you're just getting started, pregnancy fitness is not about pushing your limits. As trainer Elise Gulan says, this isn't the time to start training for the Olympics. For those who are already active, you want to maintain a healthy exercise regimen, and for those just getting started, you want to establish a safe routine. But no matter what your workout, don't get too intense about it. Relax and remember that working out during pregnancy is not about losing weight and fitting into your skinny jeans. Not at all! It's about getting healthy and staying healthy.

Here are some easy-to-follow guidelines for a fit first trimester—and a safely active pregnancy.

1. Get some cardio activity three to five days per week. If you're already active, Elise suggests a mix of walking, spinning, the el-

liptical, or jogging (if you were a runner before). Just keep things shorter and a little less intense than you would have before you were pregnant—remember, that heart rate should stay below 140. If you didn't work out before, focus on walking. Start with three short walks per day, three to five days per week. Just walk around the block, if that's all you can handle at first, and try to build up to three twenty-minute walks per day.

MD MOVES: ✳ *Activities to Avoid*

While being active is *so* good for you during pregnancy, there are some things you should avoid. Talk to your doctor about all of this, but here's a general list of what to skip:

✳ Revving your heart rate above 140 beats per minute (a heart rate monitor is a great tool to have)

✳ Working out in the heat (stay away from 100-degree yoga classes and runs in the midday summer sun)

✳ Contact sports (that's right, no more tackle football . . . sorry!)

✳ Deep twists and inversions (like the kind you might do in a regular yoga class)

✳ Sports with a serious risk of falling (think skiing, snowboarding, and mountain biking—you can rip it up next year)

✳ Getting dizzy or short of breath. If this happens, stop right away. As Elise says, don't push through the pain!

2. Practice yoga at least once a week. Yoga is one of the best things you can do when you're pregnant to stay toned and strong, to strengthen your core without deep ab work, to enhance your ability to breathe your way through difficulties, and so much more! If you already practice yoga, you can keep up your normal routine during the first trimester (with a few key modifications, like avoiding deep twists, crunches, and inversions). But skip the hot yoga, and *always* let the instructor know you're pregnant, even if you're not telling people yet. She will keep your secret and suggest modifications as needed. If you've never practiced yoga, this isn't the time to hop into a ninety-minute power flow class. Start prenatal yoga and keep it up throughout your pregnancy.

3. If you're feeling yucky and need extra motivation to get moving, I totally get it. It's hard. I had to tell myself that I wasn't going to feel any better if I stayed on the couch, so (assuming I wasn't *completely* wiped out) I tried to do some sort of exercise on most days, and usually it worked! Of course, we all have days when our body is screaming at us that we need to rest—and we should listen. But on days when you just need a little extra push to get you off the couch, keep these things in mind:

* Exercise helps you sleep! Elise promises that getting exercise during the day improves your quality of sleep at night. If you're tired (and you probably are), this will make you feel so good.

✳ Exercise provides endorphins, which boost your mood and *will* help you feel better.

✳ Exercise can help to stimulate your appetite, which is great if you're nauseous.

✳ The fitter you stay during pregnancy, the easier it will be to snap back afterward. And if you start during the first trimester, you're much more likely to stick with it when the going gets tougher (and

---

MD TUNES: ✳ *First Tri Playlist*

I was used to working out and I tried to keep that up as much as I could during the first trimester, so this is the longest mix I made while I was pregnant. I picked tunes with a good rhythm that aren't as hard-core as I like when I'm really going all out. This mix is a blend of strong, upbeat songs and more mellow stuff to remind you to go easy on yourself.

"Crazy" by Gnarls Barkley
"Home" by Daughtry
"Iris" by The Goo Goo Dolls
"Cherish" by Madonna
"The Joker Mash-up With Everything I Own" by Jason Mraz and Chrissie Hynde
"Stop and Stare" by OneRepublic
"I Shot the Sheriff" by Eric Clapton
"Chasing Cars" by Snow Patrol
"Silent All These Years" by Tori Amos
"Slide" by the Goo Goo Dolls
"Drops of Jupiter" by Train
"I'm Yours" by Jason Mraz
"Hands" by Jewel

you get bigger). Don't make the mistake of letting yourself go, thinking you'll check back in and recover nine months from now. That will only make things way too hard on yourself!

Food

The beginning of my first pregnancy was defined by emotional symptoms, but the symptoms of my second pregnancy were much more physical. With Megan, I was nauseous for the first six months. Ugh. Pregnancy is a time when you're supposed to be eating a variety of superhealthy foods, I know, but most of the time I didn't want anything but Multigrain Cheerios. And for whatever reason, the smell of certain foods, like chicken, made me especially sick. I literally ran out of the makeup room at *Days* one morning because someone was microwaving a harmless chicken dish.

Poor Dave also had to put up with my weird food issues. Like I said, chicken was a particular trigger, but I didn't expect to develop an aversion to tomatoes. I asked Dave to pick up my favorite chopped salad, the one I always get, and he went way out of his way to bring it home for me one night. We settled in to watch TV together, so psyched for a cozy night at home with take-out, and I opened my salad container and almost gagged. Since Dave had made the effort to get it for me, I acted like everything was fine. I mixed in the dressing, shook it up, took a tiny bite, and then put the salad aside while pretending to watch TV. I have no idea what we were watching.

I was so distracted by the intense tomato smell (from six feet away) that I finally had to get up and put the salad in the other room where I wouldn't smell it. By then, of course, my stomach was already upset, and I was hypersensitive, so Dave's chicken pasta started tormenting me. Trying to be discreet, I covered my nose with a throw blanket to block the odor. But Dave noticed anyway and asked if I was okay. I explained and he immediately took his dish away and brought me my reliable bowl of Cheerios, saying, "Honey, you have to eat something." (It was one of the million thoughtful little things Dave did for me during my pregnancies.)

So yes, sometimes you may feel really bad. But even when you feel gross, this is a time when eating as well as possible is really, really important. Here are tips for maintaining a healthy diet during your first trimester.

1. Listen to your doctor about all the stuff you're not supposed to be eating (and drinking) for the health of your baby. I know you have to give up some fun things, but why take the risk? You'll get to have it all again soon. So skip the raw fish (I'm a sushi lover, too, and yes, it's a total bummer!), high-mercury fish (like tuna, swordfish, shark, and tilefish—but who eats tilefish, anyway?), alcohol, unpasteurized cheeses, and anything else your doctor advises you to steer clear of. She's not trying to ruin your life—she's trying to keep harmful substances away from your baby. Be sure to ask your doctor specific questions about this, too. Don't just rely on pregnancy books (like this one) for your information. For example, I love soft cheeses. And if I can't drink wine, at least I should be able

to enjoy good cheese. So I asked my doctor for specifics regarding which cheeses to stay away from, and she gave me the quick tip that most (not all, but most) cheeses made in the good ol' U.S.A. are pasteurized. If you like to visit fancy cheese shops, just tell them your concerns. They're cheese experts; they can guide you. As it turned out, I didn't have to give up my fave triple cream. Not that I eat it all the time, mind you, but you have to have some luxuries, right?

2. For now, maintain your normal calorie intake level. You don't need to be "eating for two" yet. (And even when you do, you'll need to add only about 300 calories per day. But that comes later.) It's a lot easier to keep your pregnancy weight gain at a healthy level if you don't gain excess weight during the first trimester. Talk to your doctor now about what a healthy level of weight gain is for you. For most women it's twenty-five to thirty-five pounds, but it's really an individual thing.

You may feel bloated this trimester, and you will gain a little weight, but that's due to your blood volume increasing and your uterus expanding—it's not actual baby weight yet. Women often don't gain as much weight during their second pregnancy as they did during their first. Because the first time they really *were* eating for two (ahem . . . you never need to *double* your caloric intake), but the next time around, having learned that lesson the hard way, they do a better job of moderating themselves. Of course, this is not the time to go on a calorie-restricting diet, either. Just don't mislead yourself into thinking that you need to eat more than you usually do. You don't.

3. Get plenty of calcium. Pregnancy can seriously deplete your calcium supply—your baby needs lots of calcium to build those little bones. Meg Werner Moreta, a fantastic dietitian (Dr. H from *The Biggest Loser* introduced me to her), explained to me that because calcium is a poorly absorbed mineral, it's important to spread out your intake over the course of a day. You need 800 to 1,000 milligrams per day, so you want to have three to four servings of calcium-rich foods, like plain yogurt (which has about 450 milligrams of calcium per cup), low-fat or skim milk (a cup has about 300 milligrams of calcium), broccoli (94 milligrams per cup of cooked broccoli), and almonds (75 milligrams per ounce).

4. Keep focusing on folate (or folic acid). I mentioned this as something to start thinking about well before you're pregnant. Once you become pregnant, you should keep getting at least 400 micrograms per day. Folic acid is the synthetic form of folate, and it's found in vitamins and fortified foods; folate is found in leafy greens, legumes, and many fruits (like strawberries and oranges). A good prenatal vitamin, which you should definitely be taking, will have at least 400 micrograms of folic acid, and you can keep eating folate-rich foods, too.

5. Eat as many veggies and fruits as you can. If you're going to fill up on anything, make it nutrient-packed fruits and vegetables. Get into the routine of doing that now. It's so good for you and your baby. Plus, as Meg says, if you eat more of those, you'll be less likely to binge on empty calories.

> ## MD SIPS: ✳ *Cranberry Spritzer*
>
> I love cranberry spritzers. I drank them all the time while pregnant and nursing. They feel fun and festive—somehow plain old water doesn't feel like much fun at a dinner party or restaurant—and they are so refreshing and easy. Keep the juice to *just* a splash. In a glass, combine a splash of cranberry juice with a splash of orange juice. Fill the rest of the glass up with sparkling water, add a wedge of lime, and you have a perfect "mocktail."
>
> Note: Keep in mind that sometimes sparkling waters can be high in sodium. I know, now even water is suspect. Does it ever end? Don't worry, in most cases it's fine, but do get into the habit of reading labels just to be sure. That's a good tip generally, so I'll remind you again: Always read labels so you know exactly what you're putting in your body, all the time.

Of course, you have to take all this with a grain of salt, as my mom says. Sometimes you'll crave things without much nutritional value. In my case, that craving literally came with a grain of salt—lots of salt, actually. It's such a cliché, but I *lusted* after pickles during my second pregnancy. I mean, I started salivating just thinking about them. I mentioned the craving to Jillian Michaels, trainer and fitness genius on *The Biggest Loser*, and confessed to her that sometimes I even wanted to drink the pickle juice. Her advice? Relax and eat the pickles. When you're pregnant, it's important to not get yourself all stressed out because you're having a food craving, especially when it's as simple as a few pickles.

MD SIPS: ✳ *Cucumber Mojito (Minus the Rum!)*

Here's another idea for a fun "mocktail." I got the idea from Katsuya, a restaurant in Hollywood with a great cocktail menu. It's refreshing and delicious.

Cut a lime in half and squeeze the juice into a glass. Add a teaspoon of organic cane sugar and stir it into the juice until it dissolves. Roughly tear three mint leaves and add them to the glass, then add a few slices of peeled cucumber. Lightly muddle everything together, then add a few ice cubes and top off the glass with sparkling water.

6. Practice vigilant food safety. Wash your hands thoroughly (scrub hard and sing the alphabet while you're washing) before preparing food. Wash again if you've touched raw chicken or meat or eggs, and be sure to wash any surface that those raw foods might have touched. Cook poultry, meat, and eggs thoroughly, and—as I've already mentioned—skip the raw fish for now. Don't eat anything that smells off or is past its expiration date. Avoid prepared foods from a deli counter or gourmet shop that have been sitting at room temperature for hours. Don't eat foods from restaurants that are obviously in violation of every health code in the book. These are the basics, and you should definitely talk to your doctor about food safety rules to follow.

MD EXTRA: ✳ *Nauseous much?*

Morning sickness is such a silly term. Sure, I felt sick in the morning—and the rest of the day, too. It was no fun, for me or for my costar on *Days*. Poor James. (James Scott plays EJ.) We were in a romantic scene together, and smoke had been used in a previous scene. The smell was still on set and it really affected me. It was all I could do to get through the scene, and as soon as it was over I bolted to the bathroom and threw up. Nasty! (James was quite chivalrous about the whole thing.) Pregnancy-related nausea stinks, and there's not much you can do to make it go away completely, but here are a few tips for easing the pain a bit.

✳ Sniff citrus. For me, the smell of citrus oil calmed my nausea. I found some tangerine essential oil at a health food store and kept it with me all the time. Or you could just cut a lemon in half and smell that. Try it!

✳ Keep crackers on hand all the time, even by your bed. Eating bland foods like crackers can help alleviate nausea.

✳ Eat just a little at a time. Having small bites or sips of something healthful might make the nausea go away, or at least it will help you get some nutrients into your system.

✳ Try a few sips of ginger ale.

✳ Pay attention to when you're most nauseous and when you feel okay. At those times when you feel decent, try to get down some healthy food!

✳ Sneak in nutrients. If you can stomach fruit smoothies, for example, add nutritious foods (like carrots and spinach) into the mix so you can ingest them without really tasting them.

Fashion

The first trimester isn't the most fun in terms of getting dressed. Your bump hasn't "popped" yet, so you're not going to be wearing cute maternity clothes. But you're probably feeling bloated—this is normal, because all your fluid levels go way up as soon as you get pregnant—so your regular clothes may feel snug and unflattering. Not only are you tired and nauseous, but now you have to deal with your wardrobe issues . . . great. If you're like me and you don't want people to suspect you're pregnant until you're ready to tell them—or you just don't want to walk around feeling like your clothes are too tight—there are strategies you can try. My stylist for *The Biggest Loser*, Liza Whitcraft, helped me through my whole pregnancy with style tricks, and here are some of her tips for the first trimester.

1. Wear some clothes one size up from your normal size. This works best with tailored pieces, like structured jackets and menswear-style shirts (with feminine cuts, so they have shape and definition).

2. Go for dark colors, especially on the bottom.

3. Avoid baby-doll–style tops at this point if you don't want people guessing you're pregnant.

4. Try a tunic top. It has a slim line but doesn't cling in the middle, and it hides the high-bloat areas well. Pair it with leggings or narrow jeans.

5. Wear a chunky knit, longish sweater over leggings or jeans. But don't wear one that's way too big on you—that will just make you look bigger.

6. Stay away from thin, gauzy T-shirts. Those burnout shirts are cute on the hanger but not so much on a bloated tummy. Nightmare! As Liza says, they show every single dimple. Right now sturdier fabrics (like cotton broadcloth or heavier knits) are your best bet.

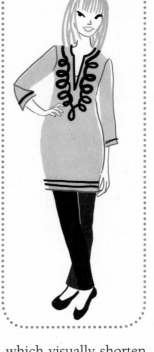

7. Show off that neckline and cleavage . . . shirts with V-necks are much more slimming than crewnecks, which visually shorten your torso. Plus, that's a part of your body that probably isn't bloated, so call attention to it.

8. In general, choose pieces that skim the body but don't cling. Baggy clothing will just make you look bigger, but that doesn't mean you should squeeze yourself into anything supertight and formfitting. Give yourself breathing room in pieces that suggest shape.

9. Remember that this is a temporary phase! Don't run out and spend a lot of money on clothes. Find a few cute and inexpen-

sive pieces that work for you, borrow clothes from a mom who's been through this or a friend who's a size larger than you are, try on what's already in your closet to see what works, and put away the stuff that doesn't make you look and feel good. Seeing it in your closet every day will just frustrate you and distract you from what fits. You will wear it again when you're ready.

Self-Care

During pregnancy, your body is working so hard and doing something really important. Plus, there's a lot of emotional work that goes into getting ready for a baby. So please, please take care of yourself while you are pregnant. It's never too early to start that! I was much better about that during my first pregnancy than my second (with two jobs and a three-year-old, it was tough), but I still tried to do what I could. Here are some simple ideas to get you into self-care mode.

1. Take naps. The first trimester can be totally fatiguing. When you feel like you can't pick your head up or get anything done, your body is telling you that you need a nap. There's nothing wrong with that. I'm not usually a nap-taker, but when I was pregnant I tried to take naps after work whenever I could. I know it's not always possible, but do it whenever you can. Baby yourself!

2. Sleep in. Hmmm, are you noticing a theme here? Sleep is so important when you are pregnant, and most women feel really

tired during the first trimester. I had less time to nap during my second pregnancy, so I tried to sleep in on weekends especially. My husband was a big help with this—he would take care of Ben so I could stay in bed. Ahhhh!

3. Chill out in comfy clothes. I'm not suggesting you spend your entire pregnancy in sweatpants. As appealing as that might sound at times, it would probably be a little depressing never to get dressed in something snazzy and go out. But when you're relaxing at home, and you don't need to worry about looking professional or anyone guessing you're pregnant, cocoon yourself in something cozy—it can still be cute, like yoga pants and your favorite T-shirt—and get really, really comfortable.

4. Start dropping hints about prenatal massages. I hate to tell you this, but as yucky as you may feel now with nausea and bloating, there's a whole new world of discomfort coming your way at the end of your pregnancy, and a good massage by someone trained to work with pregnant women can do wonders for the aches and pains. You might want one every week but that can get pricey. If your husband, mom, sister, or friends want to know what they can do for you while you're still pregnant, let them know you'd appreciate a little pampering and give them the name of your favorite spa. And set aside funds to treat yourself to at least one spa session before the big day, okay?

5. Get in the habit of asking for help. When you're pregnant, you absolutely can't do everything on your own. There will

be furniture to move and large boxes to carry, and doing it all yourself just isn't smart, healthy, or even possible. Sure, early in your pregnancy you might feel like you can still do it, but you shouldn't, and there's no better time to get used to asking for assistance. This was a tough one for me. I'm not good at asking for help at all.

One day when I was seven months pregnant, Dave came home and found that I had lodged a chest of drawers in the doorway of the baby's room. "What are you *doing*?" he demanded. "Step away from the dresser, now." Please, don't move furniture on your own, and definitely don't get anything stuck in a doorway. You need to ask for help, with everything from lifting heavy objects to cleaning the bathroom so you can nap for thirty minutes instead.

6. Take it easy on yourself if you start forgetting things or feel a little out of it mentally. You'll probably hear about a phenomenon called pregnancy brain—and it's not all in your head. Scientific studies show pregnant women and new moms are more prone to forgetfulness. It's likely hormonal—and whatever the cause, it's not your fault. Just chalk it up to "momnesia" and write things down when you really need to remember them.

7. Make time to exercise, no matter what your workout looks like these days. I know, I already talked about fitness in this chapter. But I feel so strongly that working out is a huge part of taking care of yourself. As well as helping you physically, it really lifts your spirits. It makes you feel accomplished and confident. I think there's something about all the hormones it

sets off. Try it. You'll see what I'm talking about. And if you don't set aside time to do it, you won't.

Romance

Maybe you're thinking, *Romance?! It was romance that got me into this nauseous, tired, bloated situation!* Well, you're not alone. Many women feel less than sexy during their first trimester. And some women report that their partners are a little freaked out by the knowledge of a tiny baby growing inside. The good news? Most guys get over it, and many women get a big libido boost later in pregnancy. When I was pregnant, Dave wasn't really affected sexually by the idea of it. But he did have to deal with all my new idiosyncrasies . . . like the nausea I felt before getting into bed at night. Here are some of the things you can do to get through this phase with your romantic feelings toward each other pretty much intact.

1. Cut yourself some slack. This is an adjustment period. You're getting used to being pregnant, you might not feel well, and your boobs may be sore on top of all that! Mine weren't sore in general, but they were definitely more sore in intimate situations. You need to get used to everything that's going on in your body, so don't worry if you don't feel turned on every night.

2. Communicate. Your partner can't feel what you're feeling, so you need to be open and talk about it. I had to learn to be

upfront and to let Dave know when I needed space or if I was feeling delicate in a certain area (like with my sensitive boobs), and he appreciated it when I did—because otherwise how would he know?

3. Have a sense of humor. Don't worry, your sex life isn't over if you have a few strange weeks. It's a lot more fun—and there's less pressure on both of you—if you can laugh together about any weirdness.

4. Go to an early ultrasound together. There's nothing like seeing your baby's heartbeat for the first time—or maybe a little hand—to make you feel totally in love with your partner.

5. Plan a "babymoon." Celebrate your pregnancy by booking a romantic getaway for you and your husband before the baby arrives. Plan it for when you're six or seven months along, which is when you should be feeling pretty good (over the morning sickness, and not superhuge). Make sure your doctor gives you the okay to travel. You could go somewhere you've always wanted to visit ('cause you won't have time for a while after the baby comes), but you also don't have to go far. If your doctor advises against flying or you're strapped for cash, take a short drive and have a weekend getaway nearby. You could even stay right in your own city—if you're saving on transportation expenses, you could splurge a little on a nice hotel room. Book it now and you'll have it to look forward to.

Second Trimester

Many pregnancy-related books and websites make it sound like the day after your first trimester ends, you wake up in the morning and . . . poof! No more nausea, no more fatigue, and suddenly you have the most adorable little basketball belly.

Um, sorry, that's not how it works. I'm not trying to be a buzz-kill; I just don't want you to have unrealistic expectations. For some women, the nausea does go away around the end of the first trimester, and some women never even get nauseous, but for many it goes on and on (and on . . .). With Ben my nausea went away pretty quickly, but with Megan, I felt sick and overwhelmingly tired for the first six months. I hope your nausea and fatigue go away, but I felt completely, unreasonably exhausted and ill until the end of my second trimester with my second pregnancy.

As for the cute belly? Well, as my sister-in-law says, for a while it's more like having a tire around your waist. Especially during your first pregnancy, you'll feel more pudgy than pregnant during much of your second trimester. At least now you can tell people why! If you're using this book as a refresher for a second child (which is a good idea because, believe me, I had forgotten *everything* when I got pregnant a second time, four years later), women often "pop" much earlier in their second pregnancies than they did the first time around. The good news about that is you are more obviously pregnant, so you probably won't feel you have to explain yourself as much. I guess that's the silver lining.

But wait, before you get depressed: Some amazing things happen during this trimester. Knowing that the nausea will likely go away at some point, and your pregnant belly *will* pop should be of some comfort to you. But that's nothing compared to feeling your baby move for the first time (which could happen anytime between sixteen and twenty-five weeks) and the "big" ultrasound you'll probably have around eighteen or twenty weeks. This is when you'll likely get a clear view of your baby's profile, and see its hands and so many other adorable tiny body parts . . . including (if you want) the one that tells you the baby's gender.

Not everyone chooses to learn the sex of the baby, of course, but Dave and I decided we wanted to find out. Luckily we both had the same mind-set about this decision. I have a few friends who wanted to find out but had spouses who didn't. I don't have any genius advice about how to resolve this issue except to say that you have to try to do one or the other. I'd love to say that you're the one carrying the baby, so you get to decide, but that's not fair. Yes, I know, you're doing the heavy lifting, but you're in this together . . . right? I know a few couples who decided that one of them would find out and the other wouldn't, and it was really difficult for both of them. So if you can find a way to stick together on this one, I think you'll be glad you did.

Dave was with me for both ultrasounds. It was so exciting for us to find out each time. With Ben, it was hard to see at first because he had his legs crossed for almost the whole exam, and when the technician could finally get a good look, she wouldn't tell us. But then the doctor came in, took one look, and said, "Congratulations! It's a boy."

We would have been overjoyed either way, of course. We were just so happy to know, and we actually had a boy's name picked out already. Benjamin is named after Dave's grandfather, who was an amazing man. He immigrated to the United States at the age of twelve with nothing and went on to live the American dream. Dave and his parents were very close to Grandpa Ben, and we really wanted to be able to name a child after him while he was still alive. We brought him a picture from the ultrasound and told him what the name would be, and it meant so much to us and to him.

Moments like that make all the tough parts of pregnancy much easier to bear. So hang in there!

Fitness

I know you don't want to hear this, but if you're still fighting nausea, working out can really help you feel better. Seriously, it can! I know all you want to do is lie there and feel sorry for yourself (or at least that's what I wanted to do), but if you get moving and get those endorphins flowing, that will actually help you beat those nasty feelings. And when your fatigue and nausea go away (whenever that happens), you'll probably have a stretch of weeks or months during which you have a ton of energy and feel great. With Ben, I definitely felt that way. So working out gets a little easier, for a while anyway. (Remember, though, even if you're feeling great: Don't push it and get over-heated or rev your heart rate above 140.)

But then . . . uh-oh. Just when you think you've got the hang of things and you're in a groove with your workout, the changes in your body are going to start really kicking in. Your center of gravity changes, your posture changes, and you'll probably need to adjust your workout accordingly. Also, as I got further along in my pregnancy, I became fatigued more easily when working out. So I had to adjust—and not get frus-trated by it. I used the elliptical more often and took fewer spin classes (and went to spin at times of day when the class wasn't packed). And guess what? Doing mellower workouts felt great! Here are tips for keeping up the exercise as you ex-perience the ups and downs of your second trimester.

1. Keep walking. Elise Gulan says walking is one of the best ways to get aerobic exercise throughout your pregnancy. It's great for you, but it doesn't stress your joints like running, which is especially important as you gain weight. On tired days, you can stroll around your neighborhood. For a more vigorous workout, try walking on the treadmill set at an in-cline. That's great for your booty, calves, and hamstrings, Elise says, and she reminds us that even as other parts of our bodies

are getting bigger, we can still keep our legs looking sexy! Try to walk or get some kind of aerobic exercise at least three times per week.

2. Start swimming. Or stick with it, if you're already a swimmer. Whether or not you usually swim for exercise, it is one of the best ways to get moving while you're pregnant. As you get heavier—and you will—your feet and joints take a beating. But when you get into the water you'll feel practically weightless. Heaven. Elise explains that swimming takes the compression off your spine, so it feels amazing for your back, too. There's no need to push it, and be sure you don't hold your breath for too many strokes. Just swim some easy laps, use a kickboard, or try water jogging. Swimming is great because it works out every muscle in your body and doesn't make you overheated. Bonus: Swimsuit anxiety goes away to some extent. You don't have to worry about whether your tummy is flat enough to look good in a bikini. You're pregnant! Try to work out in the water at least once a week.

3. Modify your yoga. If you've been doing regular yoga, during the second trimester you might want to try prenatal yoga—or if you want to stick with your favorite class, start being very cautious about any postures that might challenge your balance. Elise says the balance starts to get a little shaky during the second trimester—that's certainly what I experienced—so you should avoid or modify postures in which falling is a risk. (This is in addition to the modifications discussed on page 21, such as avoiding deep twists and inversions.) Haven't done any

yoga yet? Get yourself to a prenatal class! It's so good for your breathing and for developing your ability to work through physically challenging situations.

4. Work those arms with light weights (or resistance bands) and high reps. Like legs, arms are a body part that can look as hot as ever during pregnancy. For especially fabulous arms, Elise suggests focusing on the shoulders and triceps. If they looked toned, she says, the whole body looks toned. For shoulders, do shoulder presses with very light weights (one- or two-pound weights is all you need). For triceps, stand on the middle of a resistance band and hold the ends in your hands. Extend your arms behind you, then slowly bend your elbows and then extend them again.

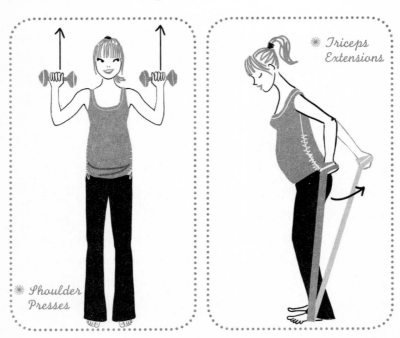

❋ Triceps Extensions

❋ Shoulder Presses

5. Develop a kegel habit (and keep it up forever). Elise explains that kegel exercises are incredibly valuable for all women, especially for pregnant women and new moms. Strengthening your pelvic floor muscles with kegel exercise can help you avoid the incontinence that can happen when the weight of your baby presses on your bladder during pregnancy; it can make birth easier, lower your risk of episiotomy, and reduce pain and swelling; it can prevent the development of hemorrhoids, increase circulation in the rectal area, and help your perineum heal from tearing; and it can increase your sexual pleasure, now and after birth. That last part alone is reason enough to do kegels!

Elise says there are many ways to do kegels; all focus on squeezing the pubococcygeus muscle (also referred to as pelvic floor muscles) repeatedly to increase strength.

Here are some variations to try—it's good to vary what you do to make your muscles stronger. Try one of these each day.

* Basic kegels: Squeeze and release the pelvic floor muscles (practice by stopping and starting the flow of urine next time you pee—that's what it feels like) up to two hundred times per day.

* Sustained kegels: Contract the pelvic floor muscles and hold for a count of ten and release. Aim for ten repetitions. If this is too intense, start with a count of five, and five repetitions, and work your way up.

* Elevator kegels: Imagine the muscles of your vagina as a building, with the base of your pelvic

MD TUNES: ✳ *Second Tri Playlist*

As I've mentioned before (yes, many times, but what can I say—I'm a big fan of yoga), if you're not already into yoga, this is a great time to start. If you don't have a good studio near you, you can buy DVDs to try at home, and if you hate the music they play as much as I do, try turning down the sound (once you understand the positions) and play your own music to motivate you. Good tunes are key to helping you get in the mood. This is my favorite yoga mix, and it's good for walking, too.

"Fix You" by Coldplay

"Flake" by Jack Johnson

"She Talks to Angels" by the Black Crowes

"Who Will Save Your Soul" by Jewel

"Like a Prayer" by Madonna

"Thank You" by Alanis Morissette

"Breathe (2 AM)" by Anna Nalick

"Hazy Shade of Winter" by The Bangles

"Hate Me" by Blue

"I'll Be There for You" by Bon Jovi

floor as the bottom floor and the top floor at your belly button. Elise says you should slowly "raise the elevator" (tighten the muscles) from the bottom floor to the top, hold for a moment, and "bring the elevator back down," slowly relaxing your muscles from top to bottom.

✳ Progressive kegels: Squeeze a little bit and hold for five counts. Squeeze a little harder and hold for five counts. Squeeze as hard as possible, and hold for another five counts. Then regress in the same manner: Release a little, hold for five counts. Release a little more and hold for five counts, then release completely. (If you're doing this one, repeat it two or three times per day or more.)

Food

For many women, myself included, food cravings really kick in during the second trimester. With Ben, I was also hungry more often—a response to the fact that you do need to start taking in some (*some*—not tons!) more calories at this point. Of course, there was less room in my belly for food because the baby was growing, so I had to eat smaller meals more often. I was always armed with healthy snacks, like almonds, low-fat granola, and energy bars, so I didn't inhale empty calories instead of eating something nutritious. Here are some tips for eating well during your second trimester.

1. Indulge your cravings from time to time. (Finally, a tip everyone can get excited about!) Unless a food you crave is on the not-during-pregnancy list (like sushi and unpasteurized cheeses), give your body what it's hungering for. Just try to be smart about it. With Ben, I craved a Fatburger every day for two weeks straight. I didn't eat one every day, mind you, but I definitely gave in to the craving more than I probably should have. That's a lesson I learned for my second pregnancy.

While I was pregnant with Ben, I hadn't started working on *The Biggest Loser* yet, so I wasn't as aware of how many calories I was actually taking in; I let myself get away with indulging a little *too* often because I was pregnant. Luckily, I gained only thirty-five pounds, which is within the guidelines for healthy pregnancy weight gain. But let's be honest—it's still a big weight gain to recover from, especially since I'm only five feet, five inches tall. But even knowing what I know now, I would have let myself have one or two Fatburgers during that pregnancy!

With Megan, I wanted candy and ice cream, even though I don't usually crave sweets. While I found a healthy way to deal with this most of the time (see number 4 on page 50), occasionally I would treat myself to a small cookie or mini-cupcake. But just one! Mini-cupcakes usually have about 100 calories, which really isn't so bad. Working on *The Biggest Loser* has taught me a lot about the calorie counts of some of my favorite (make that former favorite) foods. (See some eye-opening numbers on page 221.) It's so great to be armed with that information, for two reasons. First, now I usually have a really good sense of what I'm eating, without having to worry and calculate each and every calorie. I can just estimate pretty easily and accurately because I know the truth about what I'm consuming. Second, just knowing that those huge store-bought muffins can contain around 500 calories (yowzers!) usually prevents me from indulging. Still, I did allow myself a treat from time to time. I probably had one or two sweets a week. In between "real" treats, I fed my cravings with fruit.

Being pregnant in the summer can be great because there are so many delicious fresh fruits available. I would take Ben down

MD EXTRA: ✳ *Double Your Pleasure*

If you are pregnant with twins, wow! That is such exciting news—probably a bit shocking to you, too. When you're carrying multiples, your calorie needs increase a bit more than they do for a single pregnancy. The range of healthy weight gain is higher, too: twenty-seven to fifty-four pounds (unless you were underweight or overweight when you got pregnant). Talk to your doctor about your specific weight parameters and caloric requirements, of course, but keep in mind that you'll probably need to consume something like an extra 500 to 600 calories during your second trimester and 600 to 700 calories per day during your third trimester. You also have extra hormones floating around in your system, which could make your mood swings extra wacky and your symptoms like nausea and fatigue more intense. After you give birth, you'll have a little more weight to lose (and a little less free time to devote to getting in shape). Whew! I know that sounds like a lot to deal with, but you can do it! The good news is that people will be offering to pitch in and lend a hand more readily, knowing you have double trouble. Help yourself by staying as healthy and fit as possible during your pregnancy, following your doctor's instructions carefully, and being twice as kind and forgiving to yourself on the road to recovery. And, of course, enjoy your *two* (or more!) bundles of joy.

to the farmers' market on Sundays and pick out fresh produce to take home. I remember peaches tasting better than ever before. Once I sat down and practically inhaled half a cantaloupe before I realized what I was doing. It was so juicy and good that I couldn't stop. When Ben said, "Mommy? Can I have some?" I realized I might have polished off the whole thing without sharing. Oops.

MD EATS: ✳ *Eight Great Healthy Snacks*

One way to keep your caloric intake under control—without stressing too much—is just to eat like you normally would, and then add two or three healthy snacks during the day to give you those extra 200 to 300 calories. Nutritionist Meg Moreta gave me a bunch of easy ideas for sensible (and nutritious) things to munch on. Here are my favorites!

1. Green apple with Parmesan cheese. Yum. This is such a good combo. Cut a medium green apple into wedges and slice ½ ounce of Parmesan cheese paper thin. Have a slice of cheese with each apple wedge (about 120 calories).

2. Tomato, mozzarella, and basil. I love a Caprese salad, and this small version of it makes a very satisfying snack. Cut a medium tomato into chunks, combine it with 1 ounce of diced fresh mozzarella, add some fresh basil, and drizzle with just a bit of red wine vinegar (about 100 calories).

3. Greek yogurt with berries. This is one of my all-time favorites. Combine ½ cup of fat-free Greek yogurt with ½ cup fresh blueberries or strawberries. Sprinkle it with a little cinnamon for a different flavor (about 120 calories).

4. Medium apple with 2 teaspoons of almond butter or peanut butter. Sweet, crunchy, and satisfying! This is another favorite of mine, and very easy to prepare. Peanut butter, frankly, is a winner. It goes with so much,

⟶

is a source of protein, and is always delicious. My sister-in-law lived on PB&J sandwiches when she was pregnant, even in the middle of the night. I'm not saying that's the best idea, but sometimes you have to indulge your cravings. Just keep the amount of peanut butter you consume in check, because it is very calorie dense (about 175 calories).

5. Whole wheat mini pita with 1 ounce of feta, lettuce, and a few halved cherry tomatoes. This is a Greek salad and a pita sandwich all in one (about 135 calories).

6. Baby carrots and hummus. Grab a handful of organic baby carrots (14 to 20) and dip them in 2 tablespoons of hummus. People often use hummus as an excuse to eat chips. Don't do it. Try carrots instead. They are a great dipping food and go really well with hummus (about 100 calories; see recipe on page 52).

7. Red pepper and tzatziki. (Tza-what? See recipe on page 53.) Slice up one medium red pepper and dip the slices into ¼ cup tzatziki (about 100 calories).

8. Hard-boiled egg with a sprinkle of sea salt. This is a great source of quality protein, so it's very satisfying, and it takes care of that salt craving, too. I do it the Martha Stewart way: You put the eggs in a pot with enough water to cover them, bring the water to a boil, and then immediately turn off the heat. Let them sit, covered, for exactly 12 minutes. Works every time (about 90 calories)!

2. Add calories. But not too many! At this point, you are eating for two. Well, sort of. Your baby is getting all of its nutrition from you, but you need only 200 to 300 extra calories per day to take care of this. That's really not a lot of calories. What you need lots and lots of are nutrients, not empty calories, so focus on eating healthy foods, not calorie-dense ones.

MD EATS: ✳ *Simple Hummus*

Makes about 2 cups

Hummus is a protein-rich dip that I love to eat with baby carrots, cucumber slices, celery sticks, or slices of red or yellow bell pepper. This is a very basic recipe—you can play around with the amount of garlic and spice, or mix in diced peppers, artichoke hearts, or other veggies you think taste great with hummus.

> 1 (15- to 16-ounce) can chick-peas (aka garbanzo
>   beans), drained
> 3 tablespoons lemon juice
> 2 tablespoons water
> 1 tablespoon olive oil
> 1 garlic clove, peeled
> 1 teaspoon salt
> 1 teaspoon cumin, paprika, or your favorite hummus
>   spice
> Pepper (optional)

Combine the chick-peas, lemon juice, water, oil, garlic, salt, and spice (if using) in a food processor or blender and blend until smooth. Transfer to small bowl. Taste and season with additional salt and pepper, if desired. Keeps for up to 1 day, covered in the refrigerator.

> ## MD EATS: ❋ *Easy Tzatziki*
> ### *Makes about 1½ cups*
> Tzatziki is a traditional (and yummy and refreshing) Greek dip made mainly with yogurt and cucumbers. It's a great source of calcium, and it makes eating raw veggies more fun. It often has raw garlic in it, but I left that out of this recipe because so many pregnant women are sensitive to strong flavors and odors. But feel free to add a diced clove or two of garlic if you like.
>
> *1 teaspoon olive oil*
> *1 teaspoon lemon juice*
> *1 cup Greek yogurt*
> *½ cup diced cucumber*
> *1 teaspoon chopped fresh mint or dill (optional)*
> *Salt and pepper*
>
> In a small bowl whisk the oil and lemon juice into the yogurt. Stir in the cucumber. Season with mint or dill (if using) and salt and pepper to taste. Use as a dip for your favorite vegetables.

3. Eat your greens. Well into my second trimester I still had to force myself to eat veggies, but I found I started to enjoy things like raw spinach or lightly steamed green beans with a simple lemon vinaigrette (see recipe on page 54). If you can handle stronger flavors, try steamed broccoli or kale. Try to have green veggies at least once every day—that's a good way to get iron, fiber, and a host of other nutrients.

Tip: A fun little trick that makes salads even yummier is mixing whole herb leaves in with the greens. I had a salad like that at a restaurant and fell in love with it. So now I add cilan-

> **MD EATS: ✳ *Simple Lemon Vinaigrette***
>
> *Makes ½ cup*
>
> Give just about any green vegetable a kick of citrus (which boosts iron absorption) with this supersimple dressing.
>
> *¼ cup freshly squeezed lemon juice*
> *¼ cup extra-virgin olive oil*
> *Salt and pepper to taste*
>
> In a small bowl or liquid measuring cup whisk together the lemon juice and olive oil. Whisk in the salt and pepper and drizzle lightly over your favorite salad or steamed green vegetables.

tro leaves, parsley leaves, and other leafy herbs (think mint, basil, sage, and more). Add whatever strikes your fancy. It totally glams up a simple salad, and there's a surprise in every bite.

4. If you're craving sweets, eat fruit. Okay, yes, you've probably heard this one before. But when you're pregnant, it really works. (Most of the time, anyway.) Nutritionist Meg Moreta recommends at least two servings of fruit per day. So always try to get your sugar fix with fruit first. I have never eaten as much fruit as I did the summer I was pregnant with Megan. Peaches, watermelon, cantaloupe . . . yum! And it was satisfying in a way that candy or cake could never be, because I didn't feel guilty after I ate it.

5. Pump your iron and vitamin C. You need to get plenty of iron during pregnancy, Meg says, or you could become anemic.

Try to get it from food sources such as red meat, chicken, beans, leafy greens (another reason to eat those greens!), nuts, and seeds. Having vitamin C (from an orange or tangerine, or a small glass of orange juice) makes it easier for your body to absorb iron, so don't skip that part. Vitamin C is great for your immune system, too, which can easily become compromised in pregnant women.

6. Hydrate! Drink plenty of water. You need it. If you're tired of water, Meg suggests adding slices of lemon or orange to a pitcher of water in the fridge. Try not to hydrate by drinking juice, because that's an easy way to take in calories without realizing it. One cup of juice can easily have more than a hundred calories. (Plus, you get more nutrients if you eat a piece of fruit instead of drinking juice.)

Fashion

During my first pregnancy, I had to disguise my baby belly with my wardrobe when I was shooting scenes for *Days*. My story line did not include Sami getting pregnant, so the camera guys were using all sorts of tricks to hide me. I remember the day when my flowy top just didn't cut it anymore. I was in a scene with my costar, Bryan Dattilo, who plays Lucas on *Days*. We were in a romantic scene in Sami's bedroom, and I was walking around the room. The camera guy, Mike, sighed and leaned around from behind his camera to say, "That's not going to work. I can see you . . ." and he gestured vaguely at my torso. I got sort of defensive. "What do you mean? What do you see?" I asked. And he said, "That you're pregnant!" As I've mentioned, sometime during the second trimester you will "pop," I promise, but it might not be right away. With Ben, I was six months along before I got the basketball look; with Megan, it was five months. You pop a little earlier when it's your second or third pregnancy because your muscles don't hold it in like they did during your first. This is one of the fun parts of pregnancy—when you can enjoy the gorgeous pregnant look, but you don't feel huge and unwieldy yet. Here are some ideas for embracing your sweet Buddha belly.

1. Wear great jeans. You can wear very cool jeans throughout your pregnancy. I wore my regular jeans as long as I could; when I couldn't zip them anymore, I used a Bella Band, a stretchy fabric band that holds your jeans closed (or keeps maternity jeans in place). When your regular jeans don't work anymore, invest in—or borrow—one or two really awesome pairs of maternity jeans. Trust me: These can be the difference between feeling sexy and feeling frumpy. I like Seven maternity jeans. My friend Arianne Zucker (who plays Nicole on *Days*) loved AG and True Religion jeans when she was pregnant. And my coauthor, Christie Matheson, says she wore her Paige maternity jeans pretty much every day. Finding the right fit for you just depends on your body type, so try them on until you hit upon a pair you love.

2. Layer a long, fitted tank top or camisole under tops and sweaters. I have a long torso, so even maternity styles

weren't long enough to give me comfortable coverage as my belly grew. Adding the long layer underneath gave me confidence that I was covered and even enabled me to wear some of my non-maternity tops and sweaters for a little longer than I otherwise could have. One of my best friends bought a pack of men's medium-size tank-style undershirts from Target and wore one every day, under every outfit. She swore by them.

3. When your bump emerges, show it off! I loved it when I finally looked pregnant. As Liza, my stylist, says, celebrate it. Wear stretchy T-shirts, and maybe get one with a goofy saying, like "bun in the oven" or "baby bump," that you can wear with your fabulous jeans when you're feeling silly. (But—please—don't wear one of these every day . . . that's just too much.)

4. Remember that less is more when it comes to baby-doll tops. Many pregnant women look adorable in this flowy style that is more fitted around the chest and then flares out to the waist. Liza suggests choosing tops in this style without too much volume (there's no need to wear a tent!) and that are pretty but not too cutesy in terms of color and fabric.

5. Rock the dress-and-boots combo. This was one of my favorite outfits to wear on *The Biggest Loser* while I was pregnant. A pair of tall boots with a fitted, knee-length knit dress (not too clingy, but still body conscious, in a fairly heavy knit that drapes well over your curves) says "supersexy mama!" It

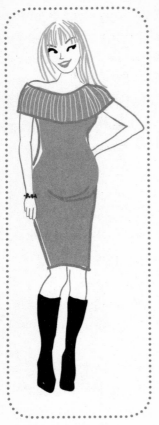

doesn't have to be an official maternity dress. My favorite was a pretty blue Juicy knit dress that I wore on *Days*. My character, Sami, was pregnant at the same time I was pregnant with Megan. (What a coincidence!) The knit was so flexible that it stretched over my belly. The fit is obviously looser now, but I still wear it and it is still flattering. I love a dress that works both ways!

6. Don't get dressed in superbaggy clothes, at least not when you go out in public. As your belly gets bigger, resist the urge (if you even have it) to hide yourself away in anything sloppy or shlumpy. That's not to say you shouldn't throw on your favorite flannel PJs, watch TV, and go to bed when you feel like it—I did plenty of that! Just try to wear pieces that are a little more body-conscious when you step out.

Self-Care

Continue to make a point of taking care of yourself—if this becomes part of your regular routine before you have a baby, you'll be more likely to stick with it after the baby arrives. You deserve it, and it's so good for you. Here are some habits to adopt now and keep forever.

1. Put your best face forward. Pregnancy can be tough on your skin. Yes, you might have that pregnancy glow (it's a real thing, from all the extra blood flow—it's awesome), but you can also develop sensitive skin and be more prone to broken capillaries. I didn't experience it, but I know some women get that pregnancy mask. Oh, and your face, um . . . fills out a bit. Here are some quick tips to try:

* You should be doing this anyway, but wear sunscreen every day. Protecting your skin from the sun makes it less susceptible to the pregnancy mask and other weird pigment things that can happen when you're pregnant.

* Use makeup, moisturizer, and makeup remover that are hypoallergenic and made for sensitive skin, with few (or no) harsh chemicals. My skin became really sensitive, and I had to make the switch from many of my usual products. La Mer skin care products, which are superpricey, are one of my splurges. If that's not in the budget, Eucerin, which is available at most drugstores, makes gentle cleansers and moisturizers that do the job well. I have a friend in New York City whose fancy Fifth Avenue aesthetician thinks Eucerin is *better* than La Mer! Christie really likes Farmaesthetics.

MD EXTRA: ✳ *A Little Help From My Friends (and Costars)*

You probably realize that your hormones can still affect your personality and emotions. I polled many mommies-to-be, and it seems that about half the time women realize in the moment that they are acting (dare I say it?) irrational, and half the time it takes some distance and perspective to see that perhaps they didn't act in quite the way they normally would. I so appreciate all the patient, supportive people who put up with my crazy mood swings during both pregnancies. It was a group effort on set. Bob, Jillian, and the contestants and crew of *The Biggest Loser* all helped me through the emotional ups and downs of my second pregnancy, and the cast and crew at *Days* helped me through both pregnancies. The guys who did the most heavy lifting were my costars, who were by my side each day on set. Bryan Datillo had become a proud father to his son, Gabriel, just a few years before Dave and I started trying to conceive. Bryan and I worked together practically every day during my pregnancy with Ben. If I got totally, irrationally upset over the smallest word in dialogue, he would calmly talk me off the ledge and help me feel better.

During my pregnancy with Megan, things were even crazier. My hormones made me feisty and quick to lose my

→

✳ Use blush (a gentle, hypoallergenic brand) to add definition and contouring to your cheeks. I also recommend, if you're naturally pale like me, using a bronzing powder to give yourself an extra boost of color. The jury's still out on whether self-tanners are safe during pregnancy, so you have to make your own decision there.

temper at the slightest provocation. I worked with Bryan Datillo and James Scott at the beginning, and I'm sure they both had moments when they wondered whether I was possessed, but managed to keep it to themselves; they were so sweet to me throughout.

Galen Gering, the proud father of two children, had just been through his wife's second pregnancy when he was cast on *Days* as Rafe Hernandez. He partnered in scenes with me (and my growing belly) almost exclusively for months. During that time, I would be fine for two weeks straight, and then one minor trigger would send me into a rage. At least I was aware that this might happen, and that it was hormonal, which helped me keep myself in check. But once I did lose it, and Galen had to sit back on the sofa in our set and watch me freak out about some little blocking detail. He then stepped in to negotiate a peace between the director and me, and afterward he was very kind as I apologized for becoming unhinged about something so minor.

If you're lucky enough to be surrounded by understanding people at work and in the rest of your life, and they help you through some of the temporary insanity of pregnancy, be sure to thank them at some point when you're feeling more like yourself!

* Wear your hair in a way that's flattering to your face. Play around to figure out what's attractive. For example, I learned that a loose ponytail with some wisps around my face looked much better than a tight ponytail. But don't do anything drastic with color or cut! (Note: These days most experts agree that coloring your hair during pregnancy is

probably safe, but you may want to talk to your doctor about this to get her opinion.) The extra fullness in your face, if you even have it, is temporary.

2. Don't worry—or beat yourself up—when strangers (or acquaintances, or relatives) start lecturing you. And they will. This is one of the most annoying aspects of pregnancy. Once people know you're pregnant, they give tons of unsolicited advice. Sure, some of it's helpful, but much of it is just the opinion of someone who thinks she (or he!) knows all the answers (but doesn't). A random woman once spotted me having a sip of Diet Coke and looked at me like I was a monster. *You're drinking that soda while you're pregnant?* Okay, lady . . . relax. People can make you feel really bad about little things if you let them—so don't let them. You know you're doing the best you can for your little nugget, so pay attention only to solicited advice from people you trust.

3. Say yes to foot rubs. You're carrying extra weight, and that puts plenty of pressure on your feet. My feet hurt a lot during both of my pregnancies, and Dave wanted to help me be more comfortable, so he offered to rub them almost every day. (Nice.) I always took him up on it.

I know that sounds like an easy thing to do, but think about it: How often do you say something like, "No, that's okay, you don't have to" when someone offers to do something nice for you? Probably too often! Consider the huge effort you are making. Nine months of pregnancy? Hello? Your hubby can handle a few foot massages, and he'll probably be happy that there's something he can do to help. (P.S. If no one is offering up foot massages to you, there's never been a better time to ask!) One note of caution: Stick to gentle rubbing and avoid the ankle-to-heel area, because it's possible that deep pressure in that area could trigger contractions.

MD EXTRA: ✳ *Be Your Own Breast Friend*

At this point you're a few months away from giving birth, and you probably haven't thought too much about what *really* happens after the baby arrives. There's no way you can truly understand what's coming, but there's one thing I'd like to tell you about now, because so many women are blindsided by it. If you plan to breastfeed your baby (and I'm not going to make a judgment one way or the other about that, but it is something I decided to try), be aware that it's not always the easiest thing to do. You've never done it before, and neither has your baby. For some women it can be quite painful. This may be an old wives' tale, but one lactation consultant I spoke with told me I could start to prepare my nipples for breastfeeding during the second trimester by scruffing them a bit in the shower with a loofah or washcloth—to build up tolerance for the forthcoming sucking, pulling, pinching, and manipulating. (Oh my.) Talk to your doctor about whether this makes sense for you and what precautions to take, because some people think stimulating the breasts can also stimulate contractions later in pregnancy. And whether you scruff or not, if you do intend to breastfeed, start prepping yourself mentally for the reality that it could be a struggle, but if it's what you want to do, it's worth it! And there are lactation consultants and products (Lansinoh Lanolin is my favorite) to help you.

4. If you get a pedicure—which I highly recommend, because it feels so good for aching feet, and it's nice to have your toes look pretty—skip the lower leg massage (just in case; see number 3, above), bring your own tools to avoid the risk of infection, and go to a place that is well ventilated and uses nontoxic polishes and removers (or bring your own). I'll be honest: I'm a bit of a germophobe. I carry hand sanitizer at all times, I don't touch public restroom doorknobs . . . you get the idea. So maybe you think this sounds over the top, but being careful about nail salons is really important, especially when you're pregnant. Choose a salon that emphasizes cleanliness, bring your own tools and healthy products, and then sit back and relax.

Romance

It can be tough to find time for romance with all the other things you're thinking about at this stage of your pregnancy. But you'll have even less time after the baby arrives. Dave and I do a lot of little things to enjoy our time together. It doesn't need to be extravagant. We love going to see movies together or just cooking dinner (I cook, he grills) and then snuggling as we watch TV together. It's important to make time for your partner and find ways to enjoy each other as a couple before you become parents. Neglecting your mutual need for romance, and physical intimacy, could put a strain on your relationship at a time when you need it to be stronger than ever, as you get ready to introduce a child into your family. Find little ways to keep the romance alive. Here are a few tips that worked for Dave and me.

1. Enjoy the simple things. Don't always try to make big romantic gestures—they're nice, but you may be too tired to pull them off. Just relish every moment together.

2. Go to the movies *now*. Dave and I saw a lot of movies while I was pregnant with Ben. When I was pregnant with Megan, we couldn't because we were busy with our then three-year-old. But with your first pregnancy, you can go whenever you want. Everyone says this because it's so true—unlike when it's hard to justify paying a sitter just to go to the movies. And by the third trimester, you aren't exactly feeling comfortable in the theater seating. Squirming and shifting in your seat when you're almost nine months pregnant is no fun, and it will likely annoy those around you. So enjoy the movies while you can!

3. Talk to your partner about what's comfortable for you in bed. I admit that I hate talking about bedroom stuff. And I'm on a soap opera that gets pretty steamy sometimes! I had some awkward moments working at *Days*. Doing love scenes, or even hugging, while you're pregnant is weird. But hopefully it's easier at home with someone you love.

Once I was shooting a scene with an actor who'd never been married and didn't have any experience with pregnant women. Our characters were supposed to be making out on a sofa, and neither of us really felt like talking about the belly bump. He started putting his weight on top of me in the scene, and I kind of panicked. I blushed beet red as I explained that it just wasn't comfortable with that kind of pressure on me, and he backed off. It was definitely one of my more awkward moments on set, but it had to be said. We found a way to balance him so that he was leaning on his side, and it worked out.

When you're with your partner, whom you know better than I knew that actor (much better!) and probably better than anyone, don't be afraid to say what's on your mind. Because then you can work through it, get past it, and get to the fun stuff. Since you're likely not supercomfortable on your back, try to let your partner know what positions you are comfortable in, and let him do more of the work.

Third Trimester

Don't be surprised if some funny things start happening to you during the third trimester. As you enter the home stretch of your pregnancy—I know, it probably seems like you've been pregnant forever, but the big day will be here before you know it—the changes in your body start to feel extreme, and your brain might get loopier and loopier, too. When I was almost nine months pregnant with both kids, I became obsessed with getting our house organized. I'd heard that the nesting instinct kicks in near the end of pregnancy, but I never thought it would happen to me. (I've always thought "nesting" is a funny concept, and I'd never had the urge before.) Well, I got the urge. Big time. During my first pregnancy, I pulled absolutely everything out of our hall closet, which was a catch-all for boxes, coats, and everything else that didn't have another place to go. We'd been throwing all our crap in there for years, and I decided that we simply could not bring a baby home until that closet was totally cleaned out and organized. It took all day, and Dave came home to find me all sweaty and dusty and gross. He laughed and said, "Ah, so this is what they mean when they talk about nesting!"

Ultimately, that was a very satisfying project to finish. Other parts of the third trimester weren't so great. Like sleeping (so uncomfortable). And eating (heartburn is awful). And getting dressed (when it feels like nothing fits anymore).

But then the moment comes when you go into labor. Now, no matter how ready you are, you'll have a moment of denial. Like, this isn't really happening, is it? And then it will hit you: Yes, it is happening . . . now! And everything else leading up to that point, no matter how difficult, sort of fades away because you're about to have the baby you've been waiting for. (Oh yeah, and deal with the whole labor and delivery thing—no sweat, right?) But until that point, you need to get through the trials and tribulations of the third trimester, so I hope this chapter can guide you through some of the tough stuff, help keep you motivated to keep exercising and eating well, and remind you to take care of yourself. This isn't easy, but you're almost there.

Fitness

It's no surprise that the bigger you get, the more difficult exercise gets. I definitely felt unwieldy. And fatigue—which usually comes back big-time in the third trimester—doesn't make it any easier to work out. But please stick with it as much as you can, even if you need to take it nice and slow. It's so good for you, and it will make your life easier both during and after delivery.

There's no need to be a hero about it, though. Sure, I know women who kept going to spin class right through the end of pregnancy. That was not me! Mostly I walked, rode the recumbent bike, and spent a little time on the elliptical, at a modified pace. I also did arm workouts with light weights. And that's about it. Here are tips for staying active as you approach your due date.

1. Keep doing cardio three to five times per week. Walking and swimming continue to be great ways to get your cardio fix. Elise Gulan also suggests workouts that let you sit down, like the recumbent bike or a rowing machine, or slow stair climbs. Make sure when you're doing cardio, you are always able to carry on a conversation. (Okay, maybe not when you're swimming, but that's the intensity level you're aiming for.) It's a simple way to monitor yourself and make sure you're not pushing too hard.

2. When working out, always, always, always drink plenty of water! And have water with you at all times. Christie learned this in a very scary way. She went for an easy jog one morning early in her third trimester and didn't drink enough water, then literally passed out in the car an hour later. Luckily, her husband was driving, but they were both completely freaked out. Even if you're just doing strength training, drinking water helps to flush out the toxins. So stay hydrated, please!

3. For strength training, avoid heavy weights and machines. Do prenatal yoga, use resistance bands, and for your lower body try moves that use your own body weight, such as lunges and wall squats. The hormone relaxin, which your body is producing to help your pelvis open up to deliver the baby, puts your muscles, tendons, and ligaments at risk of overstretching and injury if you try to lift anything too heavy. (Remember that—seriously: Always ask for help when moving or lifting something.)

LUNGES: From a standing position, step forward with one leg two or three feet. Begin bending your front knee until it is directly over your ankle (don't extend it farther than that). As you bend the front knee, lift the heel of the back leg and bend the back knee as you slowly lunge down. Stop when both knees are bent at 90-degree angles. Return to the starting position and repeat on the same side, or alternate sides.

WALL SQUATS: Stand with your back, head, and shoulders flat against a wall and your feet one to two feet away from the wall. Keeping your abs engaged, carefully lower yourself into a seated position (though you won't be sitting on anything!), adjusting your feet as needed so that your thighs are parallel to the ground and your knees are directly above your ankles. Hold for ten seconds, and repeat, or build up to holding for thirty seconds, then one minute.

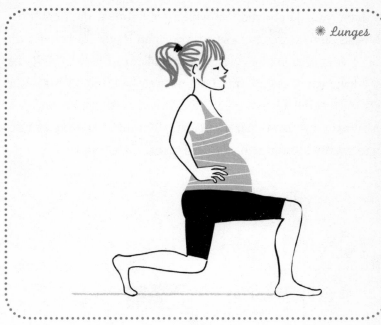

✻ *Lunges*

✻ *Wall Squats*

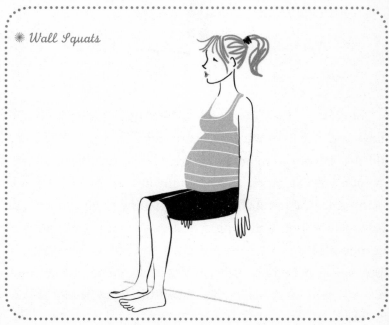

4. Shape your booty and strengthen your core at the same time with this simple exercise: Get on your hands and knees, and lift one of your legs behind you so it's parallel to the floor. Lift it a *just* a few inches, being careful not to strain or crunch your lower back, then bring it back to parallel. (This is a subtle movement—but subtle movements can be amazing for sculpting muscles.) Do ten to twenty lifts on each side, and repeat three times.

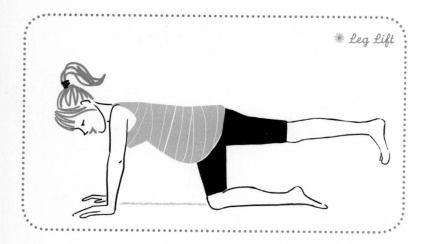

❋ *Leg Lift*

5. Think of your workout time as "me" time. It's important to allow yourself to enjoy these fairly mellow exercise sessions and just be in the moment. That's one of the reasons I love prenatal yoga so much and recommend it so strongly. It emphasizes getting in touch with and listening to your body. But really, a nice long walk would do the same thing, if you take the opportunity to be introspective and calm. My point is, don't spend the whole walk on your cell phone. Allow yourself to slow down, breathe deeply, and fully appreciate where you are.

MD TUNES: ✳ *Third Tri Playlist*

Toward the end of your pregnancy, you're going to feel uncomfortable and unwieldy. Don't beat yourself up about it . . . but don't give up on moving, either. This was the mix I listened to all the time during my third trimester. It's perfect for mellow workouts, gentle stretching, yoga on your own, and relaxed walks. It's fun to listen to, and I hope it will help you enjoy this time to get in touch with all that's happening to your body.

"Three Little Birds" by Bob Marley

"Yellow" by Coldplay

"Lay Down Sally" by Eric Clapton

"Everybody Needs Someone Sometime" by Jewel

"Meet Virginia" by Train

"(Sittin' on) The Dock of the Bay" by Otis Redding

"Accidentally in Love" by Counting Crows

"Thank You" by Dido

"Every Day I Write the Book" by Elvis Costello & the Attractions

"The Remedy (I Won't Worry)" by Jason Mraz

"How to Save a Life" by The Fray

Food

By the time the third trimester rolled around, even during my pregnancy with Megan (when I felt sick for so long), I was ready to eat again! Food was finally appealing to me, and I was hungry all the time. But it's never as easy as it should be—I couldn't eat very much at one time. There's just not much room for food, and I had terrible heartburn, especially if I ate too much at once. So I stuck to frequent small meals and tried to be as healthy as possible. Here are some guidelines for eating during the home stretch.

1. Help your immune system. While you're pregnant, your immune system is compromised. And during the third trimester, sleeping—one of the most important things you can do for a strong immune system—is so uncomfortable that it's hard to get enough. Nutritionist Meg Moreta says it's really important to bolster your immune system with food. The easiest way to do that is to keep eating at least two servings of fruit and three servings of vegetables every day. Make sure to include some vitamin C–rich foods, such as oranges, tangerines, tomatoes, kiwis, leafy greens, cruciferous vegetables (broccoli, cauliflower), berries, and red peppers. And keep taking that prenatal vitamin.

2. Keep calories under control. Yes, you're probably feeling hungrier these days, but you really need only an extra 300 calories per day at this point. Be realistic about how many calories you're taking in. For example, acknowledge that a smoothie is a meal, not a low-calorie drink. If you're buying that smoothie from a smoothie shop, it can contain upward of 500 calories.

3. Avoid heartburn. Heartburn is a condition that doesn't sound like a big deal—until you've got it. Ugh. It is *so* uncomfortable. I kept an industrial-size bottle of TUMS on the set

with me. And Meg gave me these suggestions for eating wisely to prevent heartburn:

* Really space out your meals. Eat six or seven very small meals (around 300 calories each) per day instead of three big meals.

* Have a little protein and some carbohydrates with each meal.

* Keep the last meal of the day very light.

* After your last meal before bedtime, don't just go lie down! Stay sitting up as much as possible, or— even better—go for a short walk.

* Eat only till you feel 80 percent full, and then stop. Even if you think you could eat more, don't. Chances are you'll feel full in fifteen minutes. (This is a good tip to follow all the time!)

* If you're really heartburn-prone, avoid spicy foods and caffeine, and even chocolate, which contains caffeine. Sorry!

4. Take in plenty of fiber. Yet another complaint many pregnant women have is constipation. Fun, right? Because levels of the hormone progesterone increase when you're pregnant, your digestive system slows down. As the baby gets bigger (and there's less room for everything else in there), it usually gets worse. And if you're taking iron supplements, you might get even more stopped up. Help keep things moving with reg-

MD EATS: ✳ *More Easy, Healthy Snacks*

Not only do you need to be eating about 300 extra calories per day, you want to make sure you're getting all those calories in small meals and snacks throughout the day to help you avoid heartburn (and to avoid feeling like you're *starving*). Here are some more of my favorite snacks.

HOMEMADE TRAIL MIX. It's easy to make yourself. Combine nuts (e.g, peanuts, almonds, walnuts, pecans, or cashews) and some dried fruits (e.g, raisins, cut-up dried apricots, and dried cranberries). You can put a few M&Ms in there if you need to, but I think the cranberries are sweet enough. I love the salty-sweet combo. It's a great on-the-go snack—but remember, it's calorie-dense, so you need to eat only a handful at a time.

TURKEY ROLL-UPS. Roll up one or two deli-style turkey slices with one slice of low-fat cheese, maybe a few slices of avocado, and a dollop of mustard. No bread or tortilla needed.

POPCORN. Who doesn't love popcorn? While I was pregnant, Dave taught me to make my own real pop-

→

ular exercise, plenty of water, and fiber-rich foods. Jesse Brune, a chef and trainer I work with, recommends whole grains every morning, fruits with edible skin (think apples and pears and berries), lots of veggies, and chick-peas.

5. Have a little fish. You should still be avoiding the big, mercury-laden fish such as tuna. But fish like wild salmon

corn instead of relying on the microwave brands. Now you can find 100-calorie microwave popcorn bags, which will do in a pinch, but I prefer Dave's version: Using a large pot with a lid, pour in enough safflower oil just to cover the bottom of the pot. Heat the oil over medium heat. When you think it's hot, toss one kernel of corn into the pot. When it pops, the oil is hot enough. Add 2 tablespoons of kernels and keep shaking the pot back and forth, with the lid on (crack the lid occasionally to let steam escape so the popcorn doesn't get mushy). Keep going, continuing to shake the pan, until the popping slows down. Then immediately take the popcorn off the heat and pour it into a bowl. If you mist the corn *very* lightly with water (or butter, but that adds fat and calories), salt and other seasonings will cling to the kernels and give you great flavor with every bite.

LOW-FAT STRING CHEESE. It's another great to-go snack, and when I was pregnant with Megan, I already had it in the fridge for Ben!

and sardines are rich in omega-3 fatty acids (specifically DHA, ALA, and EPA), which are key for your baby's development. You can have up to twelve ounces per week of doctor-approved fish. Walnuts and flaxseeds are good sources of ALA, while fish is the prime source of DHA and EPA.

6. Don't get freaked out by a single big jump in weight. Look at the overall picture, and if you're gaining a healthy amount

overall, you're fine. But if your doctor says your weight is creeping up faster than she'd like, take a good look at what you're eating and consider totally eliminating those occasional cupcake and cookie splurges, and filling up on veggies instead. And at every meal, think about whether you're getting the nutrients you and your baby need. Do it for yourself and for your baby. Your baby can't control what you eat, but you can!

Fashion

Okay, there's no question that you're pregnant at this point! You've definitely popped. The challenge now is finding clothes that are comfortable. I'll be honest—I dress up so much for work that when I wasn't working, I wore Juicy sweatpants and T-shirts pretty much all the time. Stretchy T-shirts that show off your belly are still supercute. It's a look that goes over well in L.A., and it didn't feel restrictive or tight on me. That's the key at this point— getting dressed in whatever makes you feel and look good!

1. Don't go out and spend much money on tons of new clothes when you have only a month or two of pregnancy left to go. You are in a temporary phase. Borrow a few maternity pieces from friends—and "pay it forward": lend clothes to girlfriends who are pregnant after you.

2. Have fun by picking up one or two (*just* one or two!) inexpensive, fun, trendy tops or dresses from someplace like Target or Old Navy.

3. Even with things you borrow and those trendy items (and definitely with anything you spend more money on), keep the cuts and colors simple: avoid loud or busy prints.

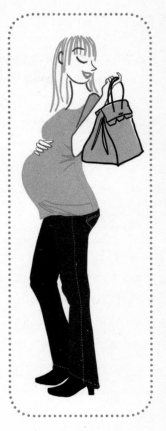

If you must splurge, do it on accessories. A great bag or a gorgeous bracelet will fit now and six months from now.

Living in L.A., I wear my flip-flops almost year round. At this stage in your pregnancy, it's really better to have shoes that support your feet. I admit that I didn't always listen to this advice myself, but I feel obligated to let you know. If your lower back starts aching, supportive shoes will really help you. That doesn't mean they have to be unattractive. If you can't give up your Chuck Taylors, and why should you, put a foot support in them to help out your back. Sneaker companies make really cute styles, too. I have New Balance tennies in black and gray that I love, and Adidas and Puma also make adorable styles in fun colors.

Self-Care

These are the last few months (for a while, anyway) that you'll be able to focus completely on you. After the baby arrives, you will be consumed with another person—a tiny, helpless, beautiful person, whom you will adore so completely you won't even mind. Still . . . you might as well enjoy a little *you* time now. It's not selfish to be selfish right now. (Remember: Taking good care of yourself means you're taking good care of your baby!)

1. Relax. Really, truly relax whenever you can. I know that's tough advice to follow because you probably have a million and one things on your to-do list. But your body is working *hard* right now, so give it a break and just chill sometimes. Everyone will understand if you miss a night out or go home early, or if you aren't the last one in the office at night.

2. If friends offer to throw you a shower, take them up on it. It doesn't have to be a long, drawn-out affair with boring games. It can be whatever you want it to be. Think of it as a nice opportunity to spend time with friends (you won't have much time for that right after the baby's born) and get little bits of good advice. Women who have babies and young children know the ropes and will give you great practical stuff that you really need. During my first pregnancy, I was lucky to have a few lovely traditional showers hosted by my family and friends. And my sister-in-law threw me a fabu-

MD EXTRA: ✳ *Pack Your Bag!*

You never know when you're going to have to rush to the hospital, and you don't need something else to think about while you're having contractions, so eliminate one reason to freak out by packing an overnight bag well in advance. I learned this the hard way—I didn't have a bag packed the first time! If that happens, the good news is that you can send someone to pick up the stuff you need. And you don't need much: I suggest a toothbrush and toothpaste and any other can't-live-without personal care products (maybe deodorant, face wash, moisturizer, lip gloss), an iPod (that was a must for me), comfy socks, clothes to wear home, and clothes for the baby to wear home. Some people recommend bringing your own pajamas, and you might want to do this, but I say use the darn hospital gown so you don't mess up your own PJs. Hospital gowns are really convenient, too, given how often you're poked and prodded and checked— not to mention nursing. One of the cutest shower gifts I got was a hospital gown made out of a really pretty feminine fabric, with ribbon trim. I wore it in the hospital with Megan, and I will admit it was a nice thing to have. Plus, it made me like the photos with my newborn that much better. One more must-have: If you'll be driving home from the hospital, you *need* a car seat. I suggest getting this (and installing the base properly) before you go into labor!

lous tea, with just a few of my closest friends. I treasured that opportunity to spend time with my girlfriends and celebrate.

When I was pregnant with Megan, my shower was held at a great place in L.A. called The Treehouse Social Club, which Joely Fisher started with her sister Trisha Leigh Fisher. It has a play area, so moms could bring their kids (no sitter required) and relax, because they knew the kids were having fun together. I loved this, because Ben could come. He enjoyed playing with the other kids, and I got some grown-up time!

3. Take time for serious pampering. Before my friend Lauren's second baby was born, instead of having a shower, three of us spent a day at a spa. We sat around in robes and drank cucumber water and got mani-pedis, and she got a pregnancy massage. By the end of the day, we were all totally relaxed. I highly recommend a day like this with a few of your pals before the baby arrives.

4. Enjoy your glowing skin. Between all the nutrients you're getting from your healthy diet and prenatal vitamins and the extra blood flow from pregnancy, your skin will really be glowing! My makeup artist, Corina Duran, suggests giving it an extra boost by exfoliating once or twice a week with a gentle scrub.

Romance

At this stage of the game, not many women really feel romantic in the traditional sense of the word. But don't let that stand in the way of having as much couple time as possible. You need that, and your husband or partner can go a long way toward

MD TUNES: ✱ *Hospital Playlists*

I made two playlists for my time in the hospital. I called one *RELAX!* and it's great for trying to zen out in a hospital bed when you hear nurse calls, announcements, and people coming to check on you constantly (or so it seems). I also had a more upbeat rock mix (*GET READY!*) for waking up and getting recharged. I wanted this one to amp me up for delivery, and I needed it to wake me up afterward, too. These are the kinds of things you generally don't think about with your first baby. It takes a trip to the maternity ward to learn how to arm yourself for a stay there. So I was much better prepared with Megan, and I was so glad to have these playlists ready to go. Hopefully you can learn some of these things from me, rather than learning the hard way.

RELAX!

"Unforgettable" by Nat "King" Cole and Natalie Cole

"Can't Help Falling in Love" by Michael Bublé

"Ol' 55" by The Eagles

"Thank You" by Dido

"Every Breath You Take" by The Police

"Only Time" by Enya

"In Your Eyes" by Peter Gabriel

"Hands" by Jewel

"Chasing Cars" by Snow Patrol

"All I Want Is You" by U2

"What a Wonderful World" by Louis Armstrong

"Ice Cream" by Sarah McLachlan

"Unchained Melody" by Righteous Brothers

"Angel" by Sarah McLachlan

"Halo" by Beyoncé

"How to Save a Life" by The Fray

"(Sittin' on) The Dock of the Bay" by Otis Redding

continued on next page →

GET READY!

"Bring Me to Life" by Evanescence

"One Week" by Barenaked Ladies

"Small Town" by John Mellencamp

"Crocodile Rock" by Elton John

"Where Is the Love?" by Black Eyed Peas

"I Gotta Feeling" by Black Eyed Peas

"Fidelity" by Regina Spektor

"Like a Prayer" by Madonna

"Shot Through the Heart" by Bon Jovi

"Pink Houses" by John Mellencamp

"Somebody Told Me" by The Killers

"Tubthumping" by Chumbawamba

"Flake" by Jack Johnson

"Won't Go Home Without You" by Maroon 5

"Accidentally in Love" by Counting Crows

"Boys Don't Cry" by The Cure

"No One" by Alicia Keys

"Proud Mary" by Creedence Clearwater Revival

"Should I Stay or Should I Go" by The Clash

"Mr. E's Beautiful Blues" by Eels

"Every Day I Write the Book" by Elvis Costello & the Attractions

"It's the End of the World As We Know It (And I Feel Fine)" by R.E.M.

bonding with the baby, through you, by taking the time to slow down and be a part of this process. So I really advise just spending as much time together as possible—comfortably, of course.

1. If you want to watch movies, I recommend NetFlix or On Demand. By my third trimester I was SUPER uncomfortable

in the theater, trying to sit through a whole movie. The heart-burn and the back pain were bad enough, and I was so self-conscious being all fidgety, knowing I was interrupting other people's movie experience. At-home movies resolve all those issues. You can pause as often as you want to go to the bath-room, or get another snack, or even watch the movie standing up if you wish.

2. When you go out, dress as comfortably as possible. This doesn't mean you can't look cute. Just don't think you need to wear four-inch heels and skinny jeans. (As if.) Christie went to a black-tie wedding when she was thirty-seven weeks pregnant, and she wore a long black knit dress (that still looked plenty dressy and chic) and left her strappy stilettos in the closet in favor of low-heeled shoes, which meant she could actually dance with her husband. She also skipped the late-night party so she could be in bed by 10:30, which ev-eryone understood.

3. Hit your favorite restaurants—the ones where you know you'll be comfortable. This is a great time to enjoy all the things you may miss for a while after the baby is born, such as a night out, a chef preparing your meal, and talking to your husband over candlelight.

4. If you have another child, spend lots of time with him and have some adventures. Dave is really good about planning fun activities for us. As we were waiting for Megan to be born, we took Ben to do some of his favorite things, like kite-flying and

going to the nearby airport to watch the airplanes take off and land. (Hey, whatever makes him happy!) We also included Ben in our discussions about baby Megan's arrival, so he was prepared for the next stage. I think it helped a lot in his adjustment to having a baby sister, and it also gave us some wonderful family memories. (This isn't a book about parenting advice, but I do suggest that if you're feeling any stress about when and how to tell an older child about a new baby on the way, ask for advice—talk to friends, preschool teachers, or your child's pediatrician about it so you feel comfortable that you're handling it appropriately.)

The First Month

For me, and for most new moms I know, the first month with a baby is all about loving this wonderful little person and trying to settle into some kind of routine. You need to figure out a feeding schedule, get some sleep, and adjust to being a parent—that's a huge adjustment. Maybe the biggest you'll ever make in your life.

During the first month after having each of my children, I didn't spend a lot of time thinking about my diet or getting my body back in shape. Okay, that's not totally true. I did spend time thinking about it. But I didn't *do* much about it! Frankly, after Ben was born, I didn't even shower for something like four days after we got home from the hospital. Gross but true.

And that's okay. It's an amazing time, and it's normal to be swept away on the new-mommy train, and to lose sight of yourself and your own goals for a while. Believe me, eventually you will shower again, and if you're anything like me, at some point, the sight of your naked body in the mirror will snap you out of your trance. And that's when you might be ready to start giving yourself the attention you deserve.

Warning: When you do first notice the state of your post-partum body, it can be frustrating. (It sure was for me.) By the end of your third trimester, you have the pregnancy "look" down. I loved emphasizing my belly and showing off what my baby-making body was able to do. But after the baby is born, the weight you gained while pregnant does not just disappear. It's still there, flopping around the gut area.

My friends all said, "It's okay! You just had a baby!" Which is true, but . . . was there a bubble over my head explaining that to every person I come across? Should I hire someone to explain that to the guy at the grocery store? People know when you're pregnant. Strangers are kinder to you; women look at you and smile as if they're sharing a secret. That all goes away after you give birth, and unless you are holding the three-week-old evidence of what your body produced, you just feel—yes, I'll say it—fat. It's not fair!

So, when you're ready, here's a gentle and easy program to follow during your first month after giving birth. No, it won't get you your prebaby body back within a few days (or weeks, for that matter). But it is a great way to start on the road to re-covery, to prepare for a more rigorous shape-up coming soon, and to help you feel good as you get used to this crazy new role you've taken on: being a mommy.

Fitness

If there's ever a time to take it easy, this is it! I know you want to get your body back, but please don't worry too much about that quite yet. You need to rest, recover, and heal—and especially if you're breastfeeding, nature will do a lot of the weight-loss work for you this month. My trainer, Stevie Sant'Angelo, says some new mommies she works with begin a walking and light hiking program as early as three weeks after having a baby, and that this can be okay for those who were active before childbirth and had a vaginal delivery. But in general, she says it's a good idea to wait until the six-week postnatal checkup to begin a real fitness regime. And that's especially true if you've had a C-section. (Talk to your doctor about what you can and can't do if you are recovering from C-section surgery.) Still, a little exercise can help fight postpartum depression and make you feel like you're somewhat in control of your body. So she suggests the following simple exercises, when you're ready, whenever you can squeeze them in, if (and only if!) your doctor says it's okay.

1. Begin with light, easy walks outside with your baby in a sling, stroller, or baby carrier.

2. Use a swill ball (also known as a Swiss ball or exercise ball—it's the big bouncy ball you often see in the abs area at the gym) and sit on it and bounce with your baby. The baby will enjoy the vertical bouncy movement and your core will be engaged the entire time, so you get a mini ab workout. (You

don't need to buy a lot of expensive equipment to follow the Mommy Diet, but I really think one of these balls—which you can get for less than twenty dollars, or borrow from a friend—is a worthwhile purchase. Check out amazon.com or sissel-online.com to find one.)

If you don't do any other exercise this month, that's fine! You're off to a great start with walking and bouncing, and it's great that you're even thinking about getting moving. But if you feel ready, and your doctor gives you the go-ahead, here are a few more simple moves Stevie suggests trying—and you can do them right at home.

3. If you have stairs, climb them two at a time with your baby in a sling or baby carrier. Or if a simple step is available (like one of your front- or back-porch steps), try sets of "step ups," stepping on and off the step, facing forward as well as sideways. Your baby is the perfect weight to challenge your body. Start with three sets of ten repetitions, then work your way up to three sets of twelve, and finally get up to three sets of fifteen repetitions. For conditioning and toning—not bulking up—fifteen reps with light weights or your own body weight is the magic number.

4. While holding a five- to eight-pound weight, try single-leg lunges forward, to the side, and backward on flat ground. Again, start with three sets of ten and work your way up to three sets of fifteen. Never increase your reps too quickly—listen to your body, do what you can, increase when you're ready, and pull it back if your form is suffering.

5. Single-leg standup: While holding two- to four-pound weights in each hand, sit on your couch or a chair. Float one leg a few inches off of the ground, and use the other leg (the one that isn't off the ground) to lift your body all the way up to standing, and then gently sit down. Keep your arms relaxed by your sides. Really try to control the movement by not wobbling the working leg. This is challenging but delivers a great-looking leg. Start with three sets of ten and work your way up to three sets of fifteen.

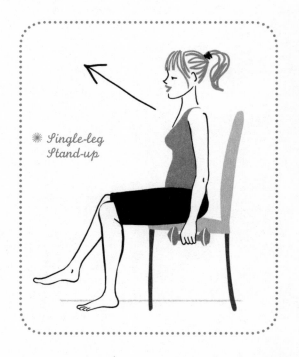

✳ *Single-leg Stand-up*

6. Triceps dips: Use a sturdy chair, couch, or weight bench. Sit down and position your hands shoulder-width apart on the front edge of the bench. Shift your body in front of the bench with your legs bent and feet placed about hip-

width apart on the floor. Slowly bend at your elbows and lower your upper body down toward the floor until your arms are at about a 90-degree angle. Keep your booty close to the bench and resist momentum on the way down. Once you reach the bottom of the movement, slowly press with your hands, and push yourself straight back up to the starting position. Keep a little bend in your elbows at the top of the movement in order to keep tension on your triceps and off your elbow joints. Make sure your chin is up; as you get stronger, straighten your legs for more of a challenge. Work up to three sets of fifteen reps.

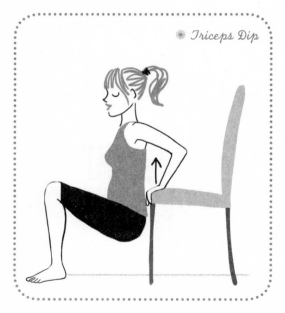

✳ Triceps Dip

7. Back stretch (this feels so good after all the nursing and bending over the bassinet or crib or changing table): If you're doing this on the swill ball—one of the few pieces of fitness gear Stevie strongly recommends investing in—have a seat

on the ball and use a towel or your hands to support your head, as you gently start to roll the ball so you can lie back over it, using your feet to "steer." Drape your body over the ball so your lower back feels well supported and your chest is opened up to the ceiling. When you're comfortable, release your hands and allow your arms and shoulders to fall where they are comfortable. Using your feet, move the ball around to find just the right position of support. (You'll know you're in the right place if your reaction is "Aaaaaaahhhh.") Recline in this position for thirty seconds to one minute a few times a day.

You can also do this on your bed: Lie down face up on your bed, positioning your upper torso so it's just a third of the way off of the bed. Using a towel or your arms to support your head, slowly drape yourself off the side of the bed. When you're comfortable, allow your arms to open up over your head and your chin to point toward the ceiling. Adjust your body position—so it's more on the bed or less—according to where it's comfortable and where you want to further your stretch. This should feel great, so if you experience any pain or discomfort, readjust your body right away. Recline like this for thirty seconds to one minute a few times a day.

Food

With everything going on in your crazy life right now, do you really have time to consider what you're eating? Well, even if you don't think so, you should try to give it a little thought. You need healthy foods to help you heal and recover from the childbirth process. If you're breastfeeding, what you eat affects your baby, so you want to eat as healthfully as possible and take in a wide variety of nutrients. And whether or not you're breastfeeding, you need healthy foods to sustain your energy and keep you feeling as good as possible during this demanding time. The good news is this: You can keep it very simple, and you don't need to be "dieting" right now.

1. Do not think about restricting calories for weight loss yet. Score! One less thing to worry about. This doesn't mean bingeing on packages of chocolate-chip cookies, but if you're breastfeeding, you need about 500 extra calories per day (that's beyond what you need just to sustain yourself) to nourish your baby. According to Stevie, that means at least 1,250 to 1,450 calories per day plus another 500, for a total of at least 1,750 to 1,950 calories. I've found that when I'm busy with a new baby, it's actually hard to get enough calories! Breastfeeding is an amazing calorie-burner, and once you're home from the hospital, where you will likely lose a good bit of weight just after having the baby, you should be losing no more than one to two pounds per week. This will happen naturally if you eat a normal, healthy diet. We will get to a more intense weight-loss diet (if you need it) in a few chapters, but for now, eat all the fruits and veggies you want and plenty of the other healthy foods you need.

MD EATS: ✻ *Supereasy Smoothie*

As Jesse says, even if you're so bad in the kitchen that you burn salad, you can make this complete meal—filled with the stuff nursing moms need—in less than a minute.

1. Take a few ice cubes from the freezer and put them in a blender.

2. Add a large handful of fresh or frozen berries.

3. Add 1 cup milk and ½ cup water.

4. Add ¼ cup plain low-fat yogurt (such as Greek-style, or your favorite kind).

5. Add 1 tablespoon flaxseed oil (optional, but a good source of omega-3s).

6. Blend for 30 seconds.

7. Drink!

2. Stock up on healthy snacks. Because you need plenty of calories, and won't have much time to eat, you'll find yourself really, really hungry at times. Be prepared with nutritious foods to munch on—easy ones, so you don't resort to devouring potato chips or Oreos. Have a friend or relative keep up your supply of fresh fruits and veggies (apples, pears, peaches, nectarines, grapes, baby carrots . . . anything you can eat on the fly). Keep small containers of yogurt, lean deli meats, string cheese, and your favorite healthy nuts (I love almonds!) ready to go whenever you need some energy.

3. Chef and trainer Jesse Brune says it's important to make sure you're consuming iron, calcium, and omega-3 fatty acids. These are superimportant right now for your health and for your baby's development.

⁕ For iron, incorporate dark, leafy greens, like spinach, into your regular food repertoire, and treat yourself to an occasional steak if you eat meat.

⁕ Drink lots of milk and eat plenty of yogurt (or find a nondairy way to get your calcium—such as more dark, leafy greens, broccoli, and calcium-fortified orange juice).

⁕ For omega-3s, eat avocados, walnuts, and about twelve ounces of fish per week, avoiding big fish like shark, mackerel, tuna, and tilefish (as you did while you were pregnant) and opting instead for safe fish like wild salmon and shrimp.

⁕ Keep taking your prenatal vitamins, especially while you're breastfeeding. Your baby is still getting her nutrition from you, so pack in those healthy vitamins and minerals.

4. Drink water. Lots of water. Your body loses a whole bunch of fluids to breastfeeding, so drink eight to ten eight-ounce glasses of water per day. (Staying hydrated can also help keep the munchies away when you're not really hungry.) Avoid caffeine as much as possible, because it's dehydrating.

MD EATS: ✳ *Month One Sample Menu*

Maybe in a month or two you'll want to try some interesting new recipes (and I have a bunch to share with you), but right now it's all about simplicity. Here's a healthy menu that will satisfy your hunger with ease.

BREAKFAST: Oatmeal or another whole-grain cereal with berries or bananas (or both) and milk

TREAT: Latte (I like tea lattes!)

SNACK: Greek yogurt and/ or fresh fruit

LUNCH: Leafy green salad with chicken or turkey

SNACK: Apple with peanut butter

DINNER: Simple roasted salmon and vegetables (For roasted salmon, heat the oven to 350 degrees F. Spray a roasting pan with cooking oil. Place a 4-ounce fillet of salmon in the pan, drizzle it with about ½ teaspoon of olive oil, season it with salt and pepper, and roast for about 15 minutes, until it flakes easily with a fork.)

5. Don't deprive yourself! Everything in moderation, right? Yes, you need to eat healthful foods right now, but if the occasional treat makes you feel better, have it. That will be good for you—and by extension, good for your baby. Little indulgences are fine if you don't go crazy. Want a cookie? Have one, not the whole bag. Craving something from Starbucks? Maybe go for the tall (that's a small) instead of the grande.

6. Before you drastically change your diet or take any supplements or restrict calories in any way, be sure to ask your doctor if it's okay.

Fashion

Okay, I know when you're tired and overwhelmed by the first few weeks at home with your new baby, being stylish isn't exactly a priority. Some days, just getting dressed feels impossible. But after hanging out in an ugly backless gown at the hospital, and probably having a few days when you never get out of your PJs, believe me when I say that taking a quick shower and getting dressed in something that makes you feel good—even if it's just putting on your favorite pink T-shirt or a pair of black yoga pants—can have a hugely positive impact on your whole outlook. Once you're somewhat settled in at home, try to get dressed every day. When you're deciding what to wear during this first month postpartum, keep in mind these tips from Liza Whitcraft:

1. Don't expect to squeeze into your old clothes right away! Too-tight clothes are never attractive, so even if you can lie down and zip up your jeans with pliers, don't. Have patience, and remember that it took you nine months to get up to the size you were when you had your baby, and it might take nine months to get back to your former size.

2. Hang on to a few of your favorite maternity pieces for a little while. Nothing tentlike, please, but maybe a great pair of jeans that look like normal designer jeans with an internal adjustable waistband, or a cute top from before you got really big. Yes, it's tempting to burn the pregnancy clothes the minute you have your bundle of joy, but some of them might help you look good and feel comfortable during the transitional first month (or two or three).

3. Skip the superbaggy clothes. Baggy clothes aren't hiding anything; they just look sloppy.

MD EXTRA: ✹ *Dress for Access!*

If this is your first time as a mom, you've probably never had to think about wearing clothes that make it very, very easy to get to your boobs. (Well, maybe you have done that before—I'm not judging!) Anyway, it's a different ball game when you're breastfeeding, and there are times when your baby will be crying and wanting to eat and all you want to do is get her to your breast. If you have to find a place to put her while you strip off a bunch of layers (or even just take off your shirt that doesn't allow for easy access), you and she may get very frustrated. So eliminate some anxiety by opting for "nursing chic" tops, like tees with crossover necklines that easily pull aside, button-front shirts, a cute cardigan over a nursing tank, and sporty zip-front jackets over nursing bras (with pads to control leakage—trust me on that) that let you get to the breast fast.

4. Wear dark colors, keep the silhouette simple, and avoid bright prints that call attention to themselves. ("Buy yourself a bouquet of flowers, don't wear it," Liza reminds me.)

5. Empire waists are still your best friends.

6. Buy two (affordable) bras at a time. Your bra size may change many times over the next few months, so don't go out and buy a dozen bras at once, but have two that fit you well right now.

7. This is still not the time to invest in expensive clothes—your current size is not permanent. Look for inexpensively flattering pieces from stores like Target, and maybe a few trendy pieces from Forever 21, or borrow some cute pieces from friends who've gone through the same transitional period. (Other moms understand—and are usually happy to help out by lending clothes or giving you hand-me-downs.)

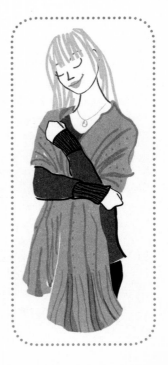

8. If you want to treat yourself to something, think about a cashmere wrap or cardigan that can cocoon you and still look good a size up from your normal size.

Self-Care

Whoa, life has changed. There doesn't seem to be much time—um, make that any time—for you these days. But as you deal with the transition from being pregnant to being a mommy, you need to find time for yourself, even if, for now, it's in increments of mere minutes. If you don't, the sheer exhaustion and feelings of being overwhelmed could easily get the better of you. Plus, your risk for postpartum depression increases if you don't get a little you time.

Now, I'm not going to tell you to book a day at the spa and take off. This month, that's just not realistic. (Don't

MD EXTRA: ✳ *Breastfeeding Comfort*

Whether you are nursing or bottle-feeding, don't forget to make yourself comfortable before getting started. I often found myself all contorted, scrunching over, trying to figure out the whole breastfeeding thing. You don't necessarily need a special breastfeeding pillow, though they are extremely helpful, but at least spend an extra few seconds adjusting pillows and positioning your back against the back of the chair or bed to make sure you are fully supported. You're going to be there for a while, and you're going to be doing this often. If you don't find yourself a comfy position, you'll end up with your back and shoulders all tense and sore. Don't make things harder on yourself. I also recommend one of those heated neck wraps. As you're getting ready to nurse, heat it up in the microwave, and then drape it over your neck and shoulders while nursing. Let the warmth soothe and relax you.

worry: There will be more pampering in the months to come.) You need to be with your baby a lot, and you'll want to be with your baby a lot. So don't feel pressure to take too much time away, but try to find little things that you can do for you. Here are a few tips—I'm talking about simple things. (Oh, you'll appreciate the simple things more than ever!)

1. Take a shower. Huh? How is that pampering? You used to do that every day, sometimes twice. Well, things are a little different now, and you might go for a few days without a shower. When you feel yourself starting to crack, hand the baby to your husband or a friend, and jump in the shower. Believe me, when you're tired, sore, and in a new-baby haze, you'll be amazed at how good it feels to have that hot water pounding on your shoulders, and to wash and rinse out your hair. You'll thank me as you're toweling off and feeling ten times better than you did before the shower!

2. Take a break! A shower is delightful, but occasionally you need to get out of the house. By yourself. Even if it's just to take a walk around the block and clear your head. The first time you do this it may feel very, very strange (both being out and about and not having your baby with you). But it's so important for your sanity. Try to do it when you know the baby has just been fed and changed. Leave your child with your hubby or someone else you trust completely, and get outside for at least fifteen minutes. During the first month, try to do this at least once every day. This is also a good trust exercise.

> **MD EXTRA:** ✳ *Stress Saver*
>
> Find the right pediatrician, and remember that no question is a stupid question when you are a new mommy. This isn't a parenting book, so I won't tell you what to look for in a pediatrician except to say find one you trust, who takes your concerns seriously no matter what they are. It will give you a lot of comfort to know that no matter what the disaster is, no matter how freaked out you get about something, your pediatrician is going to take you through each and every emergency you face as a parent calmly and coolly. This will be true till your child is a grown-up, but believe me, during this first month when everything is new, you will have a lot of things that freak you out. Reduce your stress level by calling your doctor or taking your baby in right away instead of letting your worries eat away at you. You will feel better, and sleep better, if someone has told you everything is okay—or you know what to do to fix things if there is a problem.

You and your partner *both* need to learn how to care for your new family member. You don't want to shoulder all the responsibility. Let him know he is needed and trusted in caring for your newborn.

3. Relax while you're feeding the baby. These days it will feel like you spend all your time feeding. And that's almost true—if you are breastfeeding, while your baby is still working on his efficiency, it could take forty-five minutes to an hour per session. Multiply that by eight to ten feedings a day, and we're talking up to ten hours a day feeding. Yikes! Better make those

MD EXTRA: ✸ *You're Still Beautiful Even When You're Exhausted*

This month you won't be getting much beauty sleep, or time for your hair or makeup or anything else, but there are things you can do (quickly) to combat the signs of extreme fatigue and to feel as much like your pretty self as possible. My makeup artist, Corina, is a mom herself, so it was great to be able to turn to her for advice. Here are a few things she suggests trying this month:

1. Stay hydrated! Drink tons of water. (I know, I've said it already, and you'll hear it from me again.) Aim for the eight to ten glasses a day I already recommended in this chapter. Simply drinking water can help fight the effects of stress on your skin, and though it seems counterintuitive, drinking plenty of water helps combat water retention (which you will be experiencing right now, big time). Keep your skin hydrated from the outside, too. Don't skimp on the moisturizer, and apply a hydrating mask (this takes just a few minutes) once or twice a week. I really like the hydrating products by Dermalogica and Epicuren.

2. Help your hands. You will likely be washing your hands more often than you ever have before, which can quickly dry out your skin and make your hands look about ten years older than they really are. You can avoid that easily by keeping good hand cream—one free of synthetic chemicals and fragrances or anything that might irritate your baby's skin—right next to the hand soap and applying it often. If you keep hand sanitizer around, choose a brand that's nontoxic (with no triclosan or benzalkonium chloride), such as CleanWell.

3. Exfoliate. Use a gentle exfoliant, preferably one that contains moisturizers, to brighten your skin and leave it soft.

→

4. Do your makeup in under a minute. Wearing makeup isn't an all-or-nothing proposition. It's unlikely (more like impossible!) that you'll have time for your normal makeup routine, so try using a cream blush that works for eyes, cheeks, and lips. If you don't already have this product, send a friend to buy it for you. Because it's creamy, not powdery (Corina recommends avoiding powder-based makeup right now), your skin will look fresh, dewy, and younger. Apply a little to the lips, a little to the cheeks, and a little to the eyelids, then add a swipe of mascara and you're good to go. If you have a little extra time, apply some under-eye concealer (it's a splurge, but Corina loves the concealer from Clé de Peau; Sheer Cover is a less expensive option that I like) to minimize the dark circles that are probably showing up right about now.

5. Remember that the ponytail is your friend. Don't have time to blow out your hair perfectly right now? Of course you don't! There's nothing wrong with pulling your hair back into a ponytail. It can look youthful and sporty or sleek and sophisticated or messy and sexy. Mix up the style—pull it back completely one day; pull a few pieces out to frame your face the next. Or twist the ponytail into a bun and stick the ends into your elastic (or a clip) for a do-it-yourself chignon. It's a small thing, but Juicy Couture makes hair elastics in colors with little charms on them. I love them. A touch of pizzazz in your hair might make you feel more done up to go out with no extra effort. Put on a pair of hoop earrings and you'll be amazed at how together you look. If you have short hair, run a little gel through it, part it on the side, and tuck it behind your ears for a sleek and easy look.

hours as enjoyable as possible. Often that means talking, singing, and staring at your baby. But this can be you time, too.

I love to read, and I found it really peaceful to have a book ready to read while I was nursing. (It's also nice when you're feeding with a bottle.) I suggest nothing too dense or intense. Have fun! Pick up a trashy novel or a great biography. Whatever your pleasure, take a break from being a mom for a second and catch up on reading something totally off topic. (You will be tempted to read baby care books during this time. Try not to do that constantly. You'll drive yourself nuts.) Reading non-mom material will remind you that you are more than a mother—you are a human being.

If your hands are too full to manage holding a book, set up your TV so you can watch DVR'd episodes of your favorite soap opera (of course, I recommend *Days of our Lives*). Generations of mothers have used nursing time to escape from their day-to-day issues, and they're not wrong. You have to unwind and relax when you can, even if it's while you're feeding your baby. (That's why women are the mothers. We're better at multitasking!)

4. Go out to dinner—and bring the baby! You may not be ready to leave the bambino with a sitter just yet. (If you are, go for it.) So take advantage of this time when the baby sleeps a lot and is very portable. Unless your pediatrician tells you his immune system is too compromised to go out, put him in his stroller or car seat, and go to a not-too-crowded but still lively and somewhat noisy restaurant. Make sure the baby is out of the way of foot traffic and doesn't have crowds swarming to ogle his cuteness (you don't want people sneezing on him or

spilling things on him!) and enjoy a nice meal with your husband or a good friend. At this stage, chances are the little one will sleep through the whole thing!

Romance

Be prepared: Your love life during this first month after having the baby is not going to look the same as it did before you had the baby—or, ahem, when you got pregnant. First of all, you need to give yourself time to heal. (After both vaginal and C-section deliveries, you need to allow many weeks for your whole pelvic area to rest, so follow your doctor's advice on this. I'll talk more about what happens after your doc gives you the green light for intimacy in the chapter on the second month after baby.) But physical intimacy is almost a moot point, because during this first month, both parents are just exhausted. The sheer fatigue definitely modifies your love life.

And yet it can be a really special time, and romantic in its own way. Here are some of the little things you can do to keep romance in your life this month.

1. Watch your partner bond with the baby. It is amazing to think that you have created a family together. And you've had nine months to get to know this little creature, but Dad is just meeting her for the first time. It's wonderful to see that relationship unfold and grow. Enjoy becoming a family, and remember that is a different kind of romance, but it is romantic.

MD EXTRA: ✸ *Sleep Strategies*

Say good-bye to eight straight hours of sleep at night. I'm sorry to tell you this, but this month you might be lucky if you get two or three hours in a row at any point during the day or night. This won't last forever, I promise. But until you get your baby into a sleeping routine, how are you supposed to function and feel good without a decent night's sleep?

The number one piece of advice you'll hear from people is "sleep while the baby is sleeping." It makes sense, but there will be so much you need to do in those precious moments that, realistically, there's no way you will sleep every time your baby goes down for a nap. Besides, no matter how many little naps you get during the day, for adults that doesn't make up for uninterrupted sleep. The bottom line is, when it comes to sleep, this first month is rough. Hang in there, and try these tips for getting at least a little more rest.

1. Involve your hubby with at least one middle-of-the-night feeding. If you're nursing, turn the baby over to him as soon as you're done and have him do all the legwork of burping and changing diapers and reswaddling so you can stay in a semiasleep state and go straight back to bed when the eating portion of the program is over. This won't make total sense until you are in the thick of things, but nighttime feedings are about more than feeding, and with everything else that needs to be done they can take a while. So divide and conquer!

2. Maybe you can't sleep every time the baby sleeps, but try to sleep during at least one of her daytime naps every day during this first month. Trust me, even an extra forty-five minutes or an hour of sleep in a day when you might otherwise get only three hours makes a real difference.

3. Ask for help! You know all that stuff you want to do while the baby is sleeping? Get help with as much of it as you can. That's how it's supposed to be—families used to live together, and moms would have sisters and grandmothers around to support them. Now it seems like women are determined to be supermoms and do everything themselves. I totally get that—my friends always tease me because I absolutely hate asking for help. But this is one time you have to suck it up and admit that you can't do it all by yourself. When friends offer to help you, take them up on it. Ask them to make dinner, run to the grocery store, do your laundry, or whatever needs doing so you can relax and sleep.

4. Ask for help at night, too! This one might be even tougher for the do-it-all types out there (you know who you are), but try it. Ask a family member or a close friend to stay over, once a week or every couple of nights, so that you can sleep (for as long as your body will let you if you're nursing). If you're nursing, pump a bottle for the baby, or do the feeding and then hand the baby over for all the other stuff. (This will help your husband sleep, too.) Do not wait too long to do this. I had one friend who seriously went a little crazy after several weeks of no sleep. She called me, weeping, and wasn't even aware that she was acting nuts. So a bunch of us went into helper mode and took turns relieving her during the night. I think it saved her sanity. Your close friends and family are happy to do this because they love you, so ask!

2. Say loving things to each other. I know you're tired and your patience might be nonexistent, but try not to get too crabby. You're in this together. A simple "I love you" and other sweet words mean the world right now, so remember to say them. (And let your hubby know you need to hear them!)

3. Be in touch with your partner. Literally! Holding hands, getting a back rub, a sweet kiss before you fall asleep—all of that reminds you both that you are still connected and still in love. Even if you don't have the time or energy or medical clearance to get hot and heavy, you're still there for each other. This month, even if it seems hard because you're so tired and overwhelmed, make the effort to connect with your partner—you'll both be glad you did!

The Second Month

Hey, you've made it through a whole month of being a mommy. Please take a moment to feel proud of yourself. I mean it!

During the first month after the baby is born, you do what you can to be healthy, but things are so crazy that it's hard not to be in a daze most of the time. You're trying to master changing diapers and to figure out feeding and catch some sleep, and there is no routine to speak of—you're at your baby's service, on demand.

Believe it or not, things will start to settle down (at least somewhat) in the next month or two. Your baby will likely figure out the difference between day and night and sleep for slightly longer stretches when it's dark out. The baby might not sleep through the night for a while yet, but you can begin to develop some kind of routine.

Hopefully, you will start to feel a bit more like your old self and realize that you would like to spend some time taking care of yourself. This is a good thing! I've found that many of the women who become contestants on *The Biggest Loser* are moms who never heeded their inner voice that was saying, "Wait a minute! What about me?" And they started down an unhealthy path that led them to dangerous weight gain.

I realized several years ago that if I want to be around for a long time for my family, I need to take care of myself. What's more, as a parent it's your job to set a good example, and a big part of that is setting a healthy example. As parents, I believe we are obligated to eat right and be fit, so our kids can see what it takes to do this and follow our lead. There's no better time than right now to begin creating a healthy pattern for yourself—and for your family.

Fitness

At some point during your second month after pregnancy, your doctor will likely have given you the go-ahead to get back to regular exercise. If you delivered vaginally, the recovery time is shorter—maybe just two to three weeks after delivery—but if you've had a C-section, you will need to wait until after your six-week checkup. No matter how you delivered, please wait until your doctor clears you before exercising intensely. You may look like you're healed from the outside, and you may not feel any pain, but the last thing you want to do is prevent yourself from healing properly and completely. Also, when you do get clearance to return to normal exercise, remember that it takes time to get back in shape. You've got to build up strength, endurance, and stamina—and you won't get it all back this month. But it's a great time to start.

1. Make sure you have comfortable workout gear—especially a very supportive jog bra. Your old running shorts might not quite fit right yet, and for breastfeeding moms, the bras you previously wore for workouts, even those that worked for your larger-during-pregnancy breasts, might not be enough. Because your body will change a fair amount in the coming months (and you won't be breastfeeding forever), there's no need to invest in tons of clothes. But make sure you have one or two sets of workout clothes and bras that feel great.

Elise Gulan recommends Lululemon's "Ta Ta Tamer" bra for plenty of support. Christie suggests trying to exercise just after feeding or pumping, so your boobs will feel a little less cumbersome. I actually wear two bras when I know I'm going to run or do jumping jacks or something like that. There's nothing worse than getting to the gym, pumped for a good workout, and not being able to push yourself because your bra isn't supporting you enough.

If you've never had to worry much about breast support, you may be scratching your head wondering what I'm talking about. Let me tell you, four or six weeks is not a lot of time to adjust to your new body—and your new chest size. It will feel different when you start working out vigorously again. Though this isn't a permanent state, if you don't have at least one good, ultrastrength, supportive bra, spend the money on one to make sure you don't have any excuses regarding your fitness.

2. Be creative about fitting exercise into your schedule. Suddenly getting to the gym or a yoga class, even if you're really motivated, is a whole lot harder than it used to be—you need

IS IT OKAY TO EXERCISE
WHILE YOU'RE BREASTFEEDING?

The answer is YES! Of course, you should check with your doctor to make sure there's no medical reason for you to avoid exercise. But for most women—despite what some old wives' tales say—exercise during the months when you are breastfeeding is perfectly healthy for you and your baby. And a recent study shows exercise can actually help prevent the loss of bone mineral density that often results from breast-feeding. Just be sure to stay well hydrated and eat plenty of nutritious foods.

to figure out who's going to take care of the baby. (At some point, you will probably look back on life before the baby and wonder why you didn't exercise all the time when it was so simple.) Warning: It is way too easy to use your baby as an excuse for not working out. Don't go there. You may not be able to get to the gym for an hour every day, but you can find ways to include exercise in your life.

Walk with the baby. This is pretty much always an option, and it's a good one. As you get stronger and healthier, get out there and go! Go for long walks, hilly walks, power walks. Both you and the baby will benefit from the fresh air, and you can burn some serious calories if you really work it. Stick to walks with the stroller for now—jogging strollers aren't recommended till your baby is at least six to eight months old, with very good head and neck control.

Try exercise videos. You can use these at home, while

the baby is sleeping. No babysitter needed, and no commute to the gym. And there are tons of options, many with ten-, twenty-, or thirty-minute workouts that you can do when you're really time crunched. There are yoga DVDs (I turn off the sound and listen to my own music), cardio DVDs, stretching DVDs, and more. If you're the type who loves fitness classes and working out with an instructor, this is an easy way to do that at home. You can order them online—no need to go to the store—or get them from Netflix or On Demand or even your local library.

It's a bigger investment than DVDs, but another stay-at-home option (that I loved when Megan was very young) is the Nintendo Wii Fit. I did the EA Sports Active 30-Day challenge, and it helped a lot in those early weeks. You can use the pre-planned workouts or customize one for what you want to do that day. It's also interactive, so it busts you when you're not squatting low enough or working hard enough. That helps when you're tempted to slack off.

Explore mom-and-baby fitness classes. Many yoga studios offer mom-and-baby yoga—you can bring your baby to the class and even learn how to do a few "yoga" moves with her. There are also group workouts like Stroller Strides and Baby Bootcamp. Also have your husband or a friend or a trusted babysitter commit to one or two regular times during the week when you can work out. If possible, avoid doing this at 6 a.m. or 8 p.m. or any time when you're likely to be exhausted. Figure out when you have the most energy, and plan it then. Check out alisonsweeney.com for more resources.

3. Say hello to your core! Ah, the core muscles. From abs to lower back, they are so important for just about everything you do. They support you while you're sitting, standing, walking, carrying your baby, playing sports, you name it. And wow, does pregnancy do a number on them, especially those abs.

If you had a normal vaginal delivery, you should hold off on ab work for at least two or three weeks postbirth. If you had a C-section, you need to wait at least six weeks. And Elise Gulan reminds all women that you need to see your doc before you start a real fitness plan of any kind, and one of the things she should check for is diastasis recti (stretching of the midline of the ab muscles). If you're diagnosed with diastasis recti, follow your doctor's orders about how to heal and recover before you even think about doing crunches.

Okay, having said all that, when you're finally ready to work on your core, be patient. It takes a long time to rebuild abdominal strength, so start slowly and be consistent. Try to do a gentle core workout for a few minutes three or four times per week. You can include these:

PLANK POSE: Basically, hold yourself at the top of a pushup. Make sure your shoulders are above your wrists, your arms are straight but not locked, and your hips are in line with the rest of your body (no sticking your booty up in the air or letting it sag to the ground).

Start by holding the posture for ten seconds, concentrating on tightening and strengthening your core, and slowly build up to thirty seconds and then a minute.

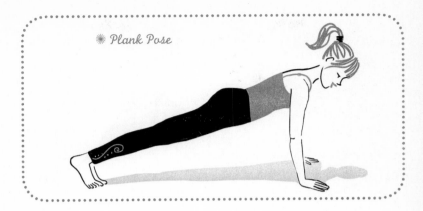

* Plank Pose

AB CURLS: Lie on your back with your knees bent and your feet on the floor. Your spine should be in a neutral position—not rounded or arched. Place your hands gently behind your head (don't use them to pull your head up) with your elbows pointing to the side. Using *only* your abdominal muscles, slowly curl your upper back off the floor, keeping your eyes on the ceiling and your head and neck relaxed and neutral (don't scrunch your chin into your chest). Curl just until your upper back is off the floor and your abs are fully engaged, then very slowly, using your abdominal muscles, lower your upper back to the floor. Start with one set of ten ab curls and slowly build up to three sets of twenty.

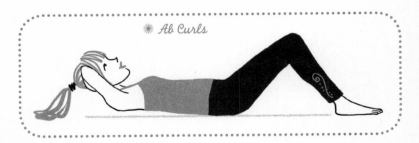

* Ab Curls

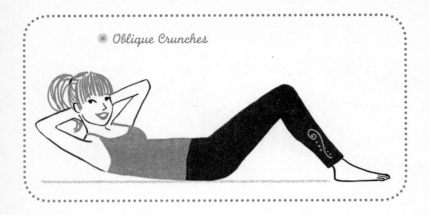

※ *Oblique Crunches*

OBLIQUE CRUNCHES: Set up as if you were doing ab curls, but then after your upper back is off the floor, use *only* your abdominal muscles (engaging your oblique abdominals, along the sides of your body) to twist your right elbow toward your left knee. *Do not* use your arms or neck or shoulders—just your abs. You don't need to touch your elbow to your knee; just twist enough to engage your obliques. Start with one set of ten on each side and slowly build up to three sets of twenty.

PELVIC TILTS: Lie on your back with your knees bent and your feet on the floor, with your arms alongside your body, palms down. Slowly and with control, engage your abdominal muscles as you tilt your pelvis toward the ceiling. This is a subtle movement; your butt shouldn't come very high off the floor, if it comes up at all. Then lower your pelvis slowly, keeping your core

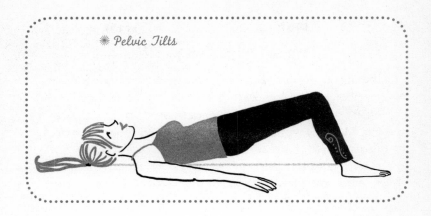

✳ *Pelvic Tilts*

muscles engaged. Start with one set of ten and slowly build up to three sets of twenty.

4. Practice yoga! This month, check out a focused postnatal class. (Many allow moms to bring their babies, as mentioned above.) This is great for full-body strengthening, and it should include gently targeted work for the abs and lower back.

5. Keep up the kegels. An important part of core work is strengthening your pelvic floor. Hopefully, you did a lot of kegel exercises while you were pregnant. And once you get clearance from your doctor, you should continue doing them. Try to get in two to three sets per day. (See a detailed description of how and why to do kegel exercises on page 45.)

> ## MD EXTRA: ✳ *Pumped Up*
>
> About a month after Ben was born, I went back to work. I remember wondering how that was going to be possible! He wasn't sleeping through the night yet, and I was breastfeeding. My body was a complete mess, especially by TV standards. Luckily, my first story line back at *Days* involved my crazy character wearing loose-fitting clothing so I was able to ease slowly back into Salem, working only a few days a week. And that was when I learned about the really glamorous world of pumping.
>
> When you pump, your body is doing what it's designed for (except there's a pump attached to your breast, and not a baby), but when I was doing it, I felt less feminine than I've ever felt. It's just not a pretty picture. Unfortunately, I really have no advice about how you can learn to like it better; I never got there. But I do have some tips on how to get through it.
>
> Not every woman's body will react the same to pumping. I have a friend who just couldn't get her body to produce very much milk that way. She was so frustrated by it but ended up discovering she needed to prompt her body by watching
>
> →

Food

Though you're on your way to figuring out this whole mommy thing, life is still pretty crazy. The idea of spending an hour in the kitchen preparing dinner probably doesn't seem feasible yet. That's okay! Keep it simple, and keep it healthy. And remember that you still don't need to be "dieting"—just focus on getting the nutrients you need and avoid overindulging in junk.

A Baby Story on TLC or other cute (happy) baby television to help her body along.

Luckily, I was able to produce plenty of milk. To help me pass the time, I bought one of those fantastic hands-free pumping bras by Easy Expressions, which made it possible for me to read a book, eat a healthy snack, or keep working at my computer if necessary. I would definitely recommend using your pumping time to take a break if you're already back at work, but that's up to you.

It can be hard to find privacy for pumping during your busy day. I know tons of moms with crazy stories about the most embarrassing place they pumped. Mine would definitely be the back of my car, in the parking lot of a charity event for St. Jude Children's Research Hospital. I was in a black-tie dress, ducking down so the parking attendant didn't see me. So please know that you're not the only one when you find yourself doing something embarrassing as a mom. Whether it's pumping in your car, or breastfeeding on the fly in public, or just wiping a snotty nose with your sleeve, it's going to happen. You're one of us now!

1. Restock your supply of easy, healthy snacks. I gave a bunch of ideas for your first month as a new mom on page 95; to add some variety this month, also try citrus fruits (like clementines, satsumas, or tangerines—the vitamin C helps with iron absorption), low-fat cottage cheese, fresh berries, pecans or cashews, two or three avocado slices, and dried fruits (try dried blueberries, cherries, and figs—or the more typical raisins, dried cranberries, and dried apricots).

MD EATS: ✳ *Ideas for Incorporating Greek Yogurt*

If you haven't caught on to this yet, I *love* Greek yogurt. It's so satisfying and creamy and healthy. I like to eat it plain, or with berries and a little cinnamon. But there are many other ways to use it. I asked chef Rocco Dispirito (who loves Greek yogurt as much as I do) for some tips on using it in all kinds of dishes. He explained that the reason we love fat-filled dairy products is because of their taste and texture. But butter contains about 1,600 calories per cup, and cream contains about 800 calories per cup. Bad news. The good news, he says, is that all-natural Greek-style yogurt (the kind without fruit on the bottom) contains just 120 to 300 calories per cup, is a great source of high-quality protein, *and* gives dishes flavor and texture similar to cream and butter. He uses it instead of butter and cream in many recipes. Here are five ways to try it:

1. Make frozen yogurt pops with just yogurt, fruit, and the healthy sweetener of your choice. Go for Stevia if you really need to cut the calories. You'll save up to 130 calories and 6 grams of fat per portion!

2. Use yogurt instead of cream in penne alla vodka (and other creamy pasta dishes) for a dramatic reduc-

→

2. If friends or relatives offer to bring food, request something healthy. Often these lovingly prepared dishes veer into fat-laden comfort-food territory (cheesy lasagna, creamy chicken pot pies), and while that's welcome early on, now you might be in the mood to lighten up a bit. Salads, soups, and whole wheat pasta salads are easy items you can suggest.

tion in calories and fat grams. You'll save up to 300 calories and 55 grams (whoa!) of fat per portion.

3. Use plain yogurt instead of cream and butter in mashed potatoes and on a baked potato. You'll save up to 350 calories and 25 grams of fat per portion.

4. Use plain yogurt instead of mayonnaise in all your dips and cold sauces. (I've also used it instead of mayo in egg salad—it was eggs-cellent. Ha.) You'll save up to 340 calories and 9 grams of fat per portion.

5. Use a mixture of plain yogurt and chicken broth as a base for your next pot pie or cream sauce. You'll save up to 500 calories and 43 grams of fat per portion.

3. Have at least one serving of yogurt per day. This is a healthy habit to adopt now and keep permanently—it gives you calcium and protein, and recent studies suggest eating yogurt daily helps with weight maintenance and healthy weight loss. Unless you're lactose intolerant, it can't hurt. (If you are lactose intolerant, try yogurt made from goat's milk, which is easier to digest.)

4. Eat soup! Sounds simple, but Meg Moreta says soup is an easy means of getting a serving or two of vegetables, and it's also warming and comforting without being too fatty (just avoid cream-based soups). Plus, it fills you up and makes you less likely to inhale something unhealthy. Soup and a salad makes a terrific, easy, healthy meal. Opt for soups with veggies, beans, lentils, and whole grains, like barley.

MD EATS: ✳ *Vegetable Curry Soup*

Serves 8

When I was hired to host *The Biggest Loser*, the producers sent me a cookbook from the show so I could understand better what I was going to be a part of. Right from the start, I loved the healthy-living message, and I loved that the books related to the show provided specific information for how to lose weight and live well on your own. I tried a bunch of the recipes, and my absolute favorite is this soup. It's so tasty, it's hard to believe it's healthy! *The Biggest Loser* said I could include it here for you all. My whole family loves this. It's totally filling as is, but sometimes I add chicken for variety.

1 tablespoon extra-virgin olive oil
1½ cups finely chopped red onion (about 2 medium)
1¼ cups finely chopped green bell pepper (about 1 large)
½ cup chopped carrot (1 medium)
½ cup chopped celery (about 2 medium stalks)
3 garlic cloves, minced
1 tablespoon curry powder
1 (14-ounce) can diced tomatoes, drained
1 bay leaf
4 cups reduced-sodium vegetable broth
½ cup cubed chicken breast meat (optional)
1½ cups (one 15-ounce can) pinto beans
¼ cup creamy or crunchy natural peanut butter or almond butter
¼ cup chopped fresh cilantro
1 (6-ounce) bag baby spinach, torn into bite-size pieces
½ teaspoon salt
Coarsely ground black pepper

→

1. Heat the oil in a 4-quart saucepan or Dutch oven over medium heat. Add the onion, bell pepper, carrot, and celery; sauté until soft and translucent, about 5 minutes.

2. Add the garlic and curry powder; sauté until fragrant, about 1 minute (do not brown garlic). Add the tomatoes and bay leaf; cook, uncovered, until the tomatoes are slightly reduced, about 3 minutes.

3. Add the broth and chicken (if using); bring to a boil. Reduce heat and simmer for about 8 minutes, until the chicken is cooked through. Add the pinto beans and peanut butter; stir to combine. Add the cilantro and spinach; cook until thoroughly heated and spinach wilts, about 2 minutes. Season with salt and pepper.

Adapted from Cheryl Forberg's recipe in Maggie Greenwood-Robinson's *The Biggest Loser: The Weight Loss Program to Transform Your Body, Health, and Life—Adapted from NBC's Hit Show!* (Rodale Books, September 2005).

Fashion

Yes, you're still recovering and sleep deprived—but hopefully you're getting out of the house more often. Putting on an outfit that makes you feel together and stylish (instead of feeling like a tired mess) can transform your outlook for a whole day. Give it a try. No need to whip out the stilettos and strapless cocktail dress. But maybe some cool jeans and a nice top will make you look and feel good.

1. Find a stylish pair of jeans that fit you now. I wore my favorite maternity jeans for a while after my babies were born. They were so comfortable, and they still looked good. But by sometime in the second month, they were just too big—I had to admit that they were starting to look sloppy. (Oh, and they were falling down, too. I knew I was really pushing it because my husband would tease me about my "gangster" look.)

Unfortunately, my prepregnancy jeans weren't yet fitting the way they used to. So I decided to find one pair of great—non-maternity—jeans that fit me during this transi-

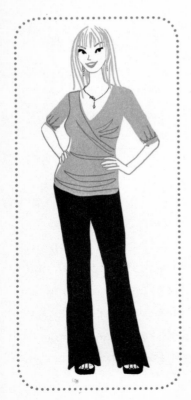

tion period, and I wore them all the time. It was so much better for my psyche than either trying to squeeze into jeans that didn't fit or resigning myself to too-big maternity wear. (The wearing-your-husband's-jeans thing? It's almost never flattering, so forget that as an option.)

Because these aren't your forever jeans, it's a good time to play with slightly trendy styles or colors—just steer clear of light colors for now. I have found that light-colored pants are only flattering on supermodels. Go for trendy, affordable styles, but remember that you're going to be happier looking in the mirror if you keep to the dark color spectrum.

2. Put together a date-night-worthy outfit that looks and feels good. And wear it one night, even if you stay home for dinner. (Hopefully, you'll wear it to go out soon, too.) Try pairing dark jeans, black pants, or a skirt with a great top with a scoop or V-neckline. Add a fun statement necklace (something with a little size and sparkle) and you're ready to go!

3. Wear cute flats. I don't know about you, but I feel much better when I'm wearing a cute pair of shoes. Heels, however, don't make a whole lot of sense this month when you'll be doing so much baby carrying. So find a great pair of flats— maybe bejeweled flip-flops or pretty ballet flats—that make you happy.

4. Put a scarf on it. It was winter (L.A. winter, but still winter!) when both my kids were born, and I became a big scarf fan. I love how they feel, and they keep my neck warm, even if I don't need a jacket here in sunny SoCal. They can also be flattering—long thin ones or long wider scarves in lightweight fabrics can create a nice long line and perhaps disguise a little tummy, too.

Self-Care

Remember you? Who? Oh, right, *you*! The mom who has learned an incredible amount in the past month, and is doing so many amazing things to care for an adorable tiny baby. The baby loves you for it (even if he can't tell you that yet), and he won't mind if you do some little things to nurture yourself for a change. In fact, if you do, you'll have much greater capacity for taking care of your beautiful little one.

1. Schedule days for sleeping in. It's not as spontaneously luxuriant as those Saturday and Sunday mornings before the baby was born, when you could sleep as late as you wanted, but at some point this month the new baby adrenaline may start to wear off, and you will need to get more sleep. Weekend mornings are a great time to squeeze in a few extra hours. Plan this in advance with your husband. Either get up to feed the baby and then head straight back to bed for some shut-eye, or have him give the baby a bottle (pump if you are breastfeeding) while you doze. Keep the door closed and the baby monitor off!

2. Share the love. At this point, hopefully you and your partner are taking turns caring for the baby. Allow your husband to play a large roll in caregiving. Because so many women are breastfeeding and "have to get up anyway," they feel the brunt of the responsibility and end up monopolizing the baby. I encourage you to share the burdens *and* the joys that go along with each stage as much as possible. You're in this together, and your husband needs baby bonding time, too.

3. Take a hot bath, and if you like it, do it once a week. Having a bath as a form of relaxation is a bit of a cliché, but there's a reason for that—it feels great. Plus, it's wonderful for the aching muscles most moms experience with all the lifting and hunching over to feed the baby. When you were pregnant you had to be careful about your core temperature, so things like hot baths and saunas and steams were off-limits (or very brief). But now you can fully enjoy them, so draw yourself a bath at home and light lots of candles (while someone else is on baby duty, of course). For extra muscle soothing and skincare, add one to two cups of Epsom salt to the tub and use a little wet Epsom salt to exfoliate your arms and legs gently before you get into the bath.

4. If you put on a top that shows off your neck and décolletage, add a little blush or bronzer around your collarbones. A little extra color and sparkle in that area can look amazing.

5. If your hair is anything like mine (which is to say it isn't supercurly, and it doesn't simply fall into place looking perfect), it's a good idea to invest in a flat iron. It definitely comes in handy when you don't have the energy to blow-dry your hair. It's a nice, easy way to give your hair a polished look. Spend the money on a good ceramic one so the heat won't damage your hair, and be sure to use a nurturing conditioner. For shine and vitality without a lot of weight, try Moroccan Oil. I love it for my hair. You can get it online at moroccanoil.com and at lots of beauty supply stores.

Romance

I think feeling "romantic" starts with feeling good about your-self. At this stage of the game, as I've mentioned several times, you are definitely tired, worn out, and maybe occasionally frustrated with your gorgeous, perfect baby. (Which is per-fectly normal and okay!) You're wondering if this phase is ever going to end, and you have trouble pulling yourself together for a trip to the supermarket, never mind a date with the man who got you into this situation in the first place. And your emotions may still be all over the place. It's totally common for women to have extreme hormonal mood swings for several months after giving birth, even if they aren't diagnosed with postpartum depression. So give yourself a break. Don't put too much pressure on yourself or heap expectations on your spouse at this time. And when you do have couple time, spend a little energy to make sure you feel the best you can about the "date." Follow my suggestions above about planning a cute outfit, do your hair, and put on a little makeup. So when you catch that last glimpse of yourself before you leave the house, you will be feeling as confident as possible . . . and that will allow you and your significant other to enjoy your time to-gether!

1. Plan a date. Even if it's just an hour long! You probably haven't had much alone time with your hubby lately. So ar-range for a friend or relative to babysit and schedule an outing—yes, please leave the house together without the baby—and enjoy yourselves. Go out to dinner, go for a walk,

go for coffee, go to an art gallery. Just pick something you both like to do—even simple activities will feel like a welcome reprieve from the baby routine, so you'll probably both be pretty easy to please when it comes to planning a date. It's perfectly fine to keep your cell phones on so the sitter can call if anything comes up. Just try not to check in every five minutes, okay?

2. Get out together for fun activities with the baby, too! You're ready to leave the house for more than doctors' appointments—and probably feeling a little stir-crazy if you haven't been going out much. So plan a hike, a walk on the beach, a picnic in the park, or a trip to a museum. Take a moment to appreciate how special it is that you are now a family unit doing things together. That's a whole new kind of romance.

3. Keep going out to dinner with the baby. He won't always fall asleep so easily and be able to sleep in his car seat for two hours straight while you eat and talk. So take advantage of this window, pick a restaurant that has a medium noise level (enough to lull him to sleep, but not loud enough to scare him), and let someone else do the cooking for you.

Months Three
Through Five

Has it happened yet? And by "it," I mean that moment when you catch a glimpse of yourself in the mirror and think, *Ugh . . . what the hell is going on with my body? Am I ever going to get rid of the rest of this baby weight? When??*

By now, you're about finished with the completely loopy brand-new baby phase, you're getting out and about all the time, and you might be heading back to work soon if you haven't already. As you return to reality, it might occur to you that you're not looking like the hottest version of yourself. And you might not love that. I had my "what the hell" moments pretty early on with both kids, because I was back to work a month after Ben was born, and ten days after Megan was born. What was I thinking?

Obviously, I was extremely optimistic when I agreed to it. I had planned my second pregnancy with the idea that I would return to work very soon after giving birth. The way the shooting schedule of *The Biggest Loser* was arranged, I wouldn't have to miss a single "weigh-in" (that's what we do at the end of each show, having each contestant step on the scale so we can find out how much weight they've lost). I knew my amazingly talented hair and makeup and wardrobe people could help me look presentable—that's what they do best. (Having Liza and Corina make me look as good as possible for work is certainly one of the very nice advantages of my profession. And they're both moms, so they knew what I was going through, and that I *really* needed their help!)

Nine-and-a-half days went by, and I was getting ready to head to the ranch to shoot. Never mind that I didn't want to be away from Megan so soon—that was harder than I ever imagined. I also felt incredibly unattractive. I felt all flabby and soft and definitely not "camera-ready," as they say. But I'd committed to going in, so I decided I had to take the plunge. And while it wasn't my most focused day of work ever, I got through it thanks to great help from the moms in my life who support me, just as I support them. Whenever your self-aware moment comes, whether it's ten days or ten weeks (or ten months) after giving birth, and you realize you want and need to get *you* back, all I can say is, I'm with you. And so is every other mom out there.

Here's what you need to know when you're having that "ugh" moment (or moments): It takes time to get your body back after having a baby. You may have heard the expression "nine months up; nine months down." As in, it takes nine months to get up to the size you are at the end of your pregnancy, and it takes nine months to get back down to your prebaby size. Every woman is different, of course, but there's some truth to this. In fact, it could take more like ten months or a year to get completely back. So please, please, please don't give up because you don't love how you look and feel yet.

I can't ask you not to be frustrated when your girlfriend bounces back from her pregnancy in no time. (I have a friend like that. I won't name names here, but let's just say I've already mentioned her in this book. She's a coworker, and we're still friends, even though she wore her prepregnancy jeans in to work her first day back, a mere seven weeks after giving birth.) I'm not a saint, and I'm guessing you aren't either, so I give you permission to mutter under your breath and think bleeped thoughts. But don't let them mess with your psyche, or your determination. You will get there, too.

And though you might not be 100 percent satisfied by four or five months postbirth, you'll be getting closer to your goals every day. You'll notice a big difference in the way you look and feel by the end of month five. Promise. So hang in there, because you're getting to where you want to be.

Fitness

Assuming you had no complications in your recovery, and you got the go-ahead from your doc to exercise several weeks or a month ago, now's the time to start making workouts a more regular part of your routine. You may not be ready for exercising five or six days per week, but during this period, let's try to work on building your stamina and endurance, exercising consistently a few days per week, and making it a little more intense as you get stronger.

1. If you're going back to work, start your childcare (at least part-time) a week before you start. This is a good idea for two reasons. First, you'll get some time for you. And second, you can ease your baby into the new routine and work out some of the kinks. During this prework week, devote some time to working out hard before the daily grind begins. Also make sure you plan some time during the work week for workouts. Maybe grab a bite on the go a few times a week and exercise during lunch. Or leave work an hour before you need to be home so you can hit the gym or a yoga class. (If you do this, please try to eat one hour before you work out. Eat something *light* and easily digestible, such as one piece of fruit or whole-grain toast with a teaspoon of peanut butter, an energy bar [under 250 calories], or a small bowl of cereal with milk. Remember when your mom said not to swim right after eating? Same thing. You don't want a nasty stitch in your side to derail your workout. You also don't want to work out with your tank on empty.) Think about this now and build it into your weekly planner. Believe me, if you don't start planning it, it's easy to let work and time with your baby completely take over your life, leaving you zero time for you. Don't let that happen.

2. If you're not going back to work, talk to other moms about forming a "babysitting club" that enables you all to have workout time. The idea is that you trade babysitting—for free—during the day. You can do this with just one other mom, or a

MD MOVES: ❋ *Sample Workout Schedule*

Here's what a week of workouts might look like at this point. Keep in mind for any ab workouts you do that you have a long road ahead of you when it comes to recovering your stomach muscles. They've been through a lot. So please don't expect to leap into an intense ab workout right off the bat. I often share the story about my first "sit-up" after having Ben—I couldn't even do one, and I literally fell back onto the ab bench at 24 Hour Fitness and laughed my head off. But you can ease yourself into it by starting early. Maybe do two or three plank poses every night before bed, for ten seconds each at first, and then build up your stamina to hold the pose for longer. As your abs grow stronger, add other ab exercises (see page 117 for ideas).

MONDAY: Day off (go for a stroll with the baby if you can)

TUESDAY: 30-minute walk-jog (warm up with a brisk 5-minute walk, then alternate 2 minutes of walking with 2 minutes of jogging for 20 minutes, then cool down with 5 more minutes of walking), plus 15 minutes of strength training

WEDNESDAY: Day off (remember to stretch in the morning or evening)

THURSDAY: 30 minutes on stair-climber or elliptical, plus 15 minutes of strength training

FRIDAY: Day off (try to walk instead of drive if you do any errands)

SATURDAY: 1-hour spin class, plus 15-minute ab workout (weekends are a great time to spend a little extra time working out—hopefully it's easier to find someone to take care of your baby on a Saturday afternoon)

SUNDAY: Day off, *or* if you want to get four workouts in this week, take a 1-hour yoga class or do something fun, like hike or play tennis

network of moms. You watch the kids for an hour or two while another mom exercises, and then she watches your little one while you work out. It's a win-win: The babies get social time, and you and your friend(s) are able to exercise without having to pay a sitter. Check out alisonsweeney.com for more ideas and an online community where you can hook up with other moms.

3. Get into a routine and develop a habit of working out at least three days per week. Up to this point, it's likely that your workouts have been sporadic. It's so amazing that you're working out at all, so please give yourself some props for that. Okay, moving on.

4. Intensify your cardio workouts. I'm not saying you need to go from leisurely strolls to hard-core sprints; just try to up the ante a bit. Going for a walk? Walk faster and add some hills. Turn the elliptical up a level or two. Increase the speed on the treadmill. Add intensity slowly, but try to push yourself a little for at least part of each workout.

5. Always have a "plan B" workout. I'm sure you've figured this out already, but as a mom, plans have a way of falling through, even when you have the best of intentions. Your number one priority is your baby, so this is okay. But don't use it as an excuse to give up on exercise. If you do that, you'll miss way too many workouts.

So if your sitter calls in sick when you were planning to go to a yoga class, pop in a yoga DVD while your baby is napping instead. Did your baby suddenly go on a bottle strike so your husband can't feed her while you're out for a hike? Don't worry, the strike will pass—for now, bring the baby and your husband hiking with you, and feed her trailside. You get the idea. Be adaptable but be firm about your need to exercise.

6. Add stretching time to your schedule. You might not have noticed how sore your muscles are, but pay attention. I'm guessing you have a few aches and pains you didn't have before. Bending over to lift an increasingly heavy baby and hunching over for feedings, not to mention getting totally out of whack with your exercise routine, take their toll on your body. So spend a few minutes gently stretching whenever you can. Ideally, you'll do it after workouts while your muscles are warm; you can also do it gently in the morning when you wake up or in the evening before bed.

I know lots of people who work out. And I would say *maybe* half of them stretch regularly. (Ahem, I am one of those people who used to forget or skip it way too often.) As a rather brutal reminder to me of my need to stretch, after a spin class, my trainer Stevie once had me lie down on my stomach while she ran a foam core cylinder over my calf muscles. She did it lightly, or so she claims, and I was literally screaming in agony. That's a little embarrassing in a gym full of people, so then I started half-crying and half-laughing through the pain, which was the result of taking too many spin classes without stretching my calf muscles afterward, Stevie explained. Her lesson worked—I now remember to stretch after every workout.

It's so good for you to stretch: It improves your flexibility, range of motion, and circulation; it might help prevent injury;

it lengthens muscles, which can help give you a long, lean look; and it feels great and helps to relieve stress in tense muscles. (You know when you're stressed out and every muscle seems tight? That's a great time for a stretching session!) Commit at least five to seven minutes to stretching and cooling down after every workout. Depending on what you concentrated on during your workout, make sure those muscles get the release they need afterward.

Here are a few of my favorite stretches:

HIPS: I love pigeon pose, a hip opener I learned in yoga class, because it hurts so good. If you know that one, try it. For a simpler hip stretch, sit on the floor with your knees bent and your feet flat on the floor a foot or two in front of you. Rest your right ankle on your left thigh, near your knee but not putting weight on your knee, so your right knee is sticking out to the side. Relax into the hip stretch. Repeat on the other side.

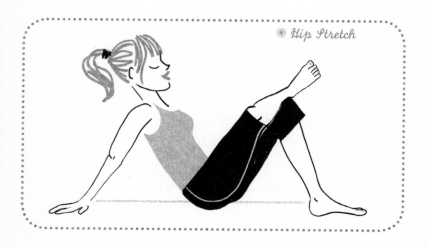

✳ Hip Stretch

BACK AND CHEST: I like to stand facing a corner, raising my arms to shoulder level and pressing my palms into the walls, to let the pressure stretch my upper back and open my chest.

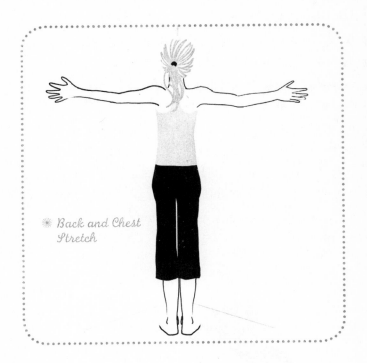

✳ *Back and Chest Stretch*

CALVES AND HAMSTRINGS: I love doing downward dog, which is a pose you know if you've done much yoga. You basically get into an upside down V. It's easiest to get there from your hands and knees. With your arms about shoulder width apart (or just a little wider), spread your fingers and press your palms and fingers (especially your thumb and index finger) into the floor, with your middle finger pointing straight ahead. Curl your toes under and push back and up, raising your hips and straightening your legs as much as you can. Keep your hips high and push them back; keep your feet about hip width apart and press your heels toward the ground. (It's okay if they don't touch—just work toward getting them closer to the ground.) Keep your arms straight (don't lock your elbows, though) and keep your back straight and neck relaxed, looking at your thighs, or the back edge of your yoga mat, if you're on one. Move your shoulders away from your ears (no scrunching) and keep your core muscles engaged. (Bonus: It's a good strengthening move, too!) You should feel a stretch in the backs of your legs, especially as you move your heels closer to the ground.

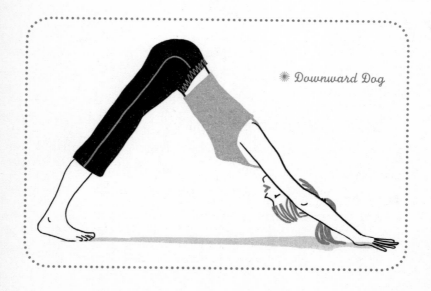

✳ Downward Dog

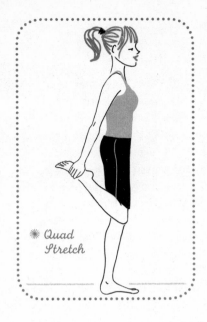

* Quad
  Stretch

QUADS: Stand up tall, with your left side facing a wall. Rest your left hand on the wall and press energetically down through the sole of the left foot. Bend your right knee and use your right hand to guide your right heel gently toward your seat until you feel a stretch, keeping your knees connected. Lengthen your tailbone downward gently and relax your hips. Hold for five to ten breaths and repeat on the other side.

Tips for safe stretching: Talk to a trainer at your gym about stretching if you've never really learned to stretch properly. Here are a few things to keep in mind—but again, if you're not sure about this, talk to a pro:

* Focus on stretching major muscle groups (calves, thighs, hips, lower back, upper back, neck, and shoulders) and especially the muscles you've been using in your workout.

* Hold each stretch for at least twenty to thirty seconds, and don't bounce!

MD EXTRA: ✳ *Stretch Anywhere!*

Think you don't have time to stretch? When I was a guest on the *Dr. Oz Show*, we discussed a few basic stretches for the glutes. I was sitting in a chair on the set, and he asked me to demonstrate by crossing one ankle over the opposite knee and simultaneously tightening my belly button toward my lap and applying gentle downward pressure with my palm to the inside of my leg (the one crossed over the other one) near my knee to increase the stretch. (This is similar to the hip stretch on page 140, but in a chair.) The stretch is only as deep as you make it, so you have control and can slowly introduce your body to the position and gradually increase your flexibility.

What I liked best about the segment, though, was that it proved you can stretch anywhere: sitting behind your desk at work, sitting on the ground watching your infant play, while watching TV, or anytime you think of it. Make it a habit to stretch whenever you can. And do some kegels while you're at it!

✳ Breathe deeply and slowly while you are stretching.

✳ Don't injure yourself. You should have that "aaah" feeling—where there's tension in that "hurts so good" way I mentioned. But if you feel real pain, back off immediately. Don't push it that far.

MD MOVES: ✳ *45-Minute Intermediate Treadmill Workout*

Looking to push yourself with a good cardio workout? Here's a 45-minute treadmill routine that will definitely get your heart pumping. It's tough, but you can do it! If you get tired, don't give up on the whole thing. Back off for 30 seconds or a minute, but *keep moving,* and try again to get back into the rhythm of the workout as soon as you're ready. Also, keep in mind that the numbers I give you here are just guidelines, and you need to do whatever is going to challenge you and get you working and sweating. And when you feel like you've mastered this one, check out the 60-minute workout on page 164!

0:00–1:30: Walk at 3.5 miles per hour, with the incline set at 2 percent. (As I mention when describing my 60-minute workout, adding a little incline gives you a more intense workout.)

1:30–10:00: Jog at 5.0 (keep the incline at 2 percent).

10:00–20:00: Do intervals, alternating between 90 seconds of hard running at 7.0 or more and then 1 minute of speed-walking (this is your active recovery period) at about 4.0. Start with the hard running and end with the speedwalking.

20:00–24:00: Slow the treadmill way down to 1.0 or 1.5 and do moving lunges.

24:00–32:00: Increase the incline to 4 percent and jog at 5.0.

32:00–40:00: Slow down to 3.0 or 3.5 speed and crank the incline way up to 10 percent. Climb that hill!

40:00–45:00: Bring the incline back down to 2 percent, and cool down with 1 minute of jogging at 5.0, 2 minutes of speedwalking at 4.0, 1 minute of walking at 3.0, and a final minute of walking slowing at 2.0. Nice job!

MD TUNES: ✳ *Favorite Workout Songs Playlist*

Looking for a new playlist to inspire you? I was, too, so I asked my Twitter fans for their favorite workout songs. Here's the list I put together based on the great ideas they tweeted.

"Beat It" by Michael Jackson

"When Love Takes Over" by David Guetta

"Let It Rock" by Kevin Rudolf (feat. Lil Wayne)

"Eye of the Tiger" by Survivor

"Animals" by Nickelback

"Stand Out" by Tye Tribbett

"Edge of Seventeen" by Stevie Nicks

"Cowboy Casanova" by Carrie Underwood

"Hips Don't Lie" by Shakira

"Super Freak" by Rick James

"TiK ToK" by Ke$ha

"Yoo Hoo" by Imperial Teen

"Ace of Spades" by Motorhead

"Toxic" by Britney Spears

"Fever" by Cascada

Food

The habits I've been encouraging you to develop and stick to—eating lots of fruits and veggies, avoiding foods you *know* are loaded with fat and calories, stocking your fridge and cabinets with healthy foods so you have them when you're hungry—still apply, and they are still the best rules to follow for effective, steady weight loss. If you're occasionally frustrated that you're not losing weight faster, maybe you're thinking it's time for a rapid-weight-loss, superpower diet. Nope! That's not the way to go for healthy and lasting results. Stick with the tried-and-true rules, and you'll get where you need to be.

1. If you're still breastfeeding, accept that you'll likely hold on to an extra five (or more) pounds of weight until you stop. Meg explained to me that this is the body's way of protecting your ability to breastfeed. So don't think you're doing anything wrong, and definitely don't cut your calories way back. Even for nonbreastfeeding women, Meg says you should never consume fewer than 1,200 calories per day, or you'll mess with your metabolism and kick your body into starvation mode (which would have an effect that's exactly the opposite of what you want—you'd start clinging to weight). So when you're breastfeeding, you need more like 1,700, minimum, and more if you're active. You can and will lose weight slowly and steadily at this rate.

MD EXTRA: ✳ *Important Weight-Loss Note*

While you're still breastfeeding, I want to emphasize again how important it is to lose weight slowly. Yes, you'll experience a rapid initial weight loss when you deliver the baby and shed fluids, but after that try to stick to one to two pounds of weight loss per week. What's nice about all this is that it takes off some of the pressure. If you lose weight too quickly, toxins stored in your body fat are released into your bloodstream and milk supply. You don't need to lose all your pregnancy weight in a few weeks. In fact, you shouldn't! Measured, steady, moderate weight loss is the healthy way to go.

2. Eat small meals (300 to 400 calories each) every three to four hours. Meg explains that this helps to keep your blood sugar stable so you don't get crazy hungry and develop major cravings—and set yourself up to eat way more than you need.

3. I mentioned earlier that it's a good idea to eat something light and healthy about an hour before you work out. For a preworkout meal, and all other meals, don't forget to chew your food. This may sound weird, but pay attention next time you're eating and see if you're chewing everything carefully. Doing so slows you down and helps you digest better. I used to have a terrible habit of scarfing my meals down in an extremely unladylike manner. Not only is that unattractive, it's not good for your digestion. Especially before going to the gym, I'm paranoid about doing anything that might cause a cramp or a stitch in my side. Eat slowly, chew each bite, and you'll set yourself up for a well-digested meal (and a pain-free workout). You'll probably eat a little less, too, because when you eat slowly, you give yourself time to feel full instead of inhaling everything on your plate when it's more than you need.

4. Don't drink your calories. You need to take in enough calories to keep your metabolism fired up, especially if you need to support breastfeeding. However, it's all too easy to take in more calories than you need if you don't factor drinks into the equation. Stick to water, sparkling water, and tea. If you're still breastfeeding you're probably not drinking much (or any) wine or caffeine, but still, even the occasional glass of vino or a

latte contributes significant calories. Here's a look at the (rather shockingly high) calorie counts of an assortment of beverages:

Starbucks plain latte (12 ounces—that's a tall, the Starbucks version of a small): 180 calories

Starbucks vanilla latte (16 ounces—that's a grande, or medium): 280 calories

Orange juice (8 ounces): 110 calories

Cranberry juice cocktail (8 ounces): 140 calories

Nondiet soda (12-ounce can): 150 calories

Red wine (5 ounces): 125 calories

Sports drinks (12 ounces): 90 calories

Eggnog (1 cup): 343 calories (I know this is a random drink that's only available one month out of the year, but it's insane how many calories are in it. I don't care how much you like eggnog—this one's never worth it. Find another way to celebrate the holidays!)

So if you were to have a glass of OJ with breakfast, a latte on your way to work, an afternoon vanilla latte treat, and a glass of red wine with dinner, you'd have consumed 695 calories in drinks alone. And if you chug a sports drink after a workout, you're drinking back a bunch of the calories you just burned. Ouch. (For more mind-boggling calorie counts, see page 221 and alisonsweeney.com.)

Fashion

Many women return to work somewhere between two and six months postbaby. Along with that comes a whole new challenge: getting dressed for work when your prebaby professional wardrobe may not fit like it used to. But you don't want to spend your workday obsessing about how you look—you need to feel confident and be able to concentrate on your job.

After Ben was born, I was involved in a crazy story line on *Days* that required me to wear men's army fatigues. The most redeeming aspect of that whole scenario was that I was able to wear those baggy clothes for almost a month when I returned to work, so I didn't feel all self-conscious about my body. I used that time to tone up and get in shape as much as I could with my schedule, and I finally returned to wearing girl-clothes and started to feel my body was my own again. I think it took about three months the first time for me to wear size twenty-nine jeans. I hung the jeans tag up in my dressing room, feeling so proud. I wasn't "done" by any means, but I was celebrating my progress.

After Megan was born, I was back on camera for both shows very quickly. And I didn't have any outlandish story lines to hide my body behind. But luckily, on *Days*, Sami had been pregnant, too. That made me feel better because my body was "in character."

Whether you're on TV or not, you always want to look your best, right? At *The Biggest Loser*, I always try to dress professionally for the weigh-ins. Finding outfits that are flattering right after childbirth isn't easy. Here are a few tips for this stage:

1. Jackets are your friends. My stylist, Liza Whitcraft, is a big fan of jackets, which she says look good even when you're carrying some extra weight because they're structured. So they look shapely even though they don't hug your shape. She suggests choosing jackets that are lined and well constructed, and making sure they are long enough at least to reach your hips. (Short jackets that don't cover the zipper of your pants are a no-no—the look is choppy and bulky.) They can be part of a suit, or you can pair them with dark jeans for a more-casual-but-still-sophisticated style.

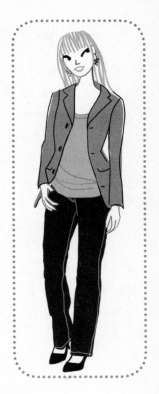

2. If you like your legs, wear skirts. For work, they should be about knee length (or just a smidge above.) Short skirts are too young looking and not professional enough for an office. Long skirts can look good if you're careful to avoid those with too much fabric and lots of pleats and gathers—I have a lightweight, wispy long skirt that I wear with a T-shirt and flip-flops; it's the perfect L.A. summer skirt—but usually they work best as part of a casual outfit. Knee-length skirts can look perfectly polished *and* show off your legs—and they tend to be more forgiving than pants around the belly, hips, and butt.

If your body is anything like mine, it's best to avoid midcalf-length skirts. They just aren't flattering to someone my height (or most anyone who's not six feet tall). Be aware of things like that: Skirts and dresses can make or break your look, depending on where the hem hits you. If you love a dress, don't be afraid to take it to a tailor and have it adjusted to the length that looks the most flattering. I was in a dress shop recently and the sales clerk offered me a 10 percent discount toward getting the dress altered at the tailor, because they want to encourage their customers to make sure the clothes fit really well. How cool is that?

3. Find a pair of great heels—about two-inch heels—that are comfy enough to wear all day. They'll add height, of course, which means you'll look slimmer and feel taller as you stride back into work.

4. For a while after my babies were born, I loved wearing tops on camera that gather in the center, right where your cleavage is, and hang down from there. It's not *too* baby doll-ish—more like a smock or trapeze top—and it drapes nicely over your belly but still shows some definition where your waist is. Velvet makes tops like this that I love.

Self-Care

Everyone is still focused on your beautiful baby at this point. Of course you understand this—you're focused on your baby, too. But when people—friends, your parents, random strangers—forget to acknowledge you with a simple *hello* because they're so eager to ooh and ah over your gorgeous progeny, you can start to feel invisible and unimportant. (You aren't. Hi!) It's easy to overlook the sense that you're being neglected, though, because that feeling is quickly masked by the pride you also feel about your baby. But this doesn't mean you should neglect yourself, too. Here are some easy ways to prioritize *you*:

1. Get to know other moms of babies around your baby's age, if you haven't already. During the first year (and beyond), talking to other moms can be one of the big keys to your sanity. They are going through the same things you are—trying to get their babies to sleep, wondering whether everything going on with their babies is normal, not having any clothes that fit quite right, husbands who want to have sex more than they do—and it really helps to be able to talk to women who completely understand where you're coming from. They can offer advice, sympathy, and simple companionship during this crazy time.

2. Spend some time with your girlfriends who don't have kids, too. Remember them? The ones you used to hang out with all the time? A little QT with these ladies can help you feel like a grown-up again. You'll laugh and have fun—if you don't spend two hours analyzing poop and sleep patterns. Keep the baby chatter to a minimum. If all your girlfriends have kids, at least spend some time with the girls while not talking about anyone under two-and-a-half feet tall.

MD EXTRA: ✳ *Hair Drying How-to*

I like playing around with different hairstyles, but I think a look that never fails for women with medium-length to long straight or wavy hair is a smooth blowout. Corina gave me these tips for blow-drying hair right:

1. After you wash and condition your hair, apply a little product to keep your hair healthy (a moisturizing product or a thermal protector). Corina likes to use a root booster for hair that needs some extra volume.

2. Rough-dry your hair to get the excess water out—your hair should be 75 to 80 percent dry when you're done with this step.

3. Divide hair into sections using clips. Working with the bottom sections first, use a round brush (the size you need depends on your hair—a bigger brush will give you more body) and move the brush through your hair, holding it taut as you dry it from the root to the end. Dry each section thoroughly before moving on to the next.

4. When all the sections are dry, apply a smoothing or shining or anti-frizz product as needed.

And here are a few other styles to try if you want to mix things up for work or a date night:

SUPERSTRAIGHT: After you blow-dry your hair straight, use a ceramic flat iron to make it as straight as you possibly can.

→

PULLED BACK: Sweep your hair away from your face into a low ponytail or twist it into a chignon (a knot pinned at the nape of your neck). You can do this with your hair straight or curly. If you have naturally curly hair, you can add a headband or a length of fabric tied at the back of your neck to keep those fabulous curls (I'm jealous) off your face.

HEADBAND: Blow-dry your hair and use a wide brush and volumizing products to give it plenty of body, then pull it back with a stylish headband.

KINDA CURLY: If your hair isn't naturally curly, don't try to fake the Shirley Temple look. Go for loose, natural-looking waves. Once your hair is dry, wrap sections of your hair around a curling iron, hold for a second, then gently pull your hair taut as you release the iron. Apply a little product with your fingers and mess up your hair just a bit.

THE "FARRAH": If your hair is cut in layers, like mine, you can do an updated "Farrah Fawcett" look. Ms. Fawcett knew what she was doing—a feathered look can be a really attractive way to frame your face. Blow your hair out as described above, and then use a large-barrel curling iron just on the ends of the layers around your face, curling them back and away from your face.

3. Do some hair maintenance. All over!

* Book a haircut, even if it's just a trim to clean up the ends a bit. (It's still not the time to do anything drastic.)

* Give your eyebrows some attention, too. Either get a professional wax or tweeze, or tweeze them yourself (working from the bottom of the brow, never the top) in very bright light.

* Shave your legs and armpits carefully and thoroughly—have you done that recently? Finally, how's that bikini line of yours? Letting that go postbaby is easy, but it's time to do something about it. Go get a bikini wax—or choose your preferred method of bikini line maintenance.

4. Take care of your scalp and your hair (I'm back to talking just about the hair on your head)—you may be losing a lot of it. Many women find their hair gets thicker and shinier than ever while they're pregnant. And then a few months after the baby is born, it starts to fall out. Like crazy. I'm talking about big handfuls coming out during every shower. Don't be alarmed, because this is normal. To protect what hair remains during the fallout phase, Corina says you should avoid using too much heat on it and damaging it. She suggests massaging your scalp with a little tea tree oil to stimulate hair growth. And use good conditioner.

5. Develop an easy prework makeup routine so you look fresh and awake, even if you didn't get a whole lot of sleep. Corina says wearing a little blush is a good idea to add color to your face, and you can sweep the blush across your eyelid, too. Add a little black or dark brown pencil eyeliner and mascara, and

try red lipstick to perk up your look. (Corina says you can't go wrong with red lipstick—you just need to use a shade of red that works with your skin tone, so try several and find the one that's right.)

Romance

Hopefully you're getting more regular sleep at night now, and feeling more like yourself. Don't beat yourself up when you're too exhausted to think, let alone be romantic. But when you're feeling good, share that with your partner!

1. Put a regular date night on the calendar. This is so important, even if you just do it once a month! I recommend getting to a point where you do it more often than that, but only you know what you can handle right now. Find a sitter you trust, or a relative willing to help out (most relatives, especially grandparents, are extremely willing). And then stick to it—yes, even on those nights when you're a little worn out. If you're totally spent, just go out for a quick bite together and then come home and go to bed. Going out as a couple is good for you both.

2. Plan "date nights" at home, too. As your baby's sleep schedule becomes more predictable, you can (I hope) start to count on a few hours or more in the evenings when the baby will be snoozing. Once a week, plan to be home together (no need for a sitter) and have a date. Eat dinner by candlelight,

watch a movie, play a game, sit and talk—whatever you're in the mood for.

3. Pick up some KY or another lubricant. Full disclosure: I am uncomfortable talking about stuff like this, but Christie *made* me put it in here. Many new moms experience discomfort and dryness when they start having sex again after having a baby (this is true whether you delivered vaginally or by C-section). Unfortunately, I think many moms are uncomfortable talking about this, like me, so you may not expect it—and it can be a surprise and a bummer. Anyway, don't be embarrassed to buy a lubricant to help you out. (It really does help.) If you're too uncomfortable to go to the pharmacy for what you need, that's what online drugstores are for. Your UPS guy will never know what's in that brown box.

4. Be aware that some guys suddenly develop an acute awareness that you're a mom—it's the "she kisses my kids with that mouth" mentality (thank you, Robert De Niro in *Analyze This*). They may be hesitant to go for it because you're a mother now. In most instances, it's just a small hurdle to overcome. Most guys aren't going to let it stop them for long. But if you're dealing with real stubbornness, again I offer my most important piece of advice for anything related to your relationship: Communication is the key. You can't let months go by with no sex, and not discuss it. You have to work through the hesitation, either yours or his, and figure out how to get past it. A physical relationship is a crucial aspect of a marriage, and it's a mistake to imagine it doesn't matter.

Shape-up Week

Less than four months after Megan was born, I was scheduled to appear on live TV for the finale of *The Biggest Loser*, which I knew millions of people would be watching. I also knew I'd have magazine photo shoots and talk show appearances. So even though I wanted to take things fairly easy and give my body the time it needed to heal, I definitely had that on my mind soon after giving birth. The truth is, it was on my mind during my pregnancy, too—and that goal did help me stay as healthy and fit as possible while I was pregnant. But after Megan was born, I really didn't stress about it for the first eight weeks, because I had a plan. I knew *Days* was going on hiatus for one week when Megan was about two months old. I didn't have to work on *The Biggest Loser* then either, so I used that week to kick-start my fitness routine.

This is something I recommend trying only when you're sure you're ready, and only when your doctor says it's okay. Pick a week and make a commitment to yourself: Eat really well, work out as often as you can (every day, if possible), and do at least one thing each day to pamper your body. You might want to plan a week like this before you return to work, or at the three- or four- or five-month mark, or prior to a wedding or another big event, or whenever it makes sense for you.

During my shape-up week I worked out every single day. Please note: This doesn't mean I did a twenty-mile run followed by three hours in the gym every day. Not even close. I was still recovering and trying to get back into shape, so I didn't want to get hurt or push myself too hard. But I did definitely intensify my workouts in sort of a bootcamp-style regime, mostly focusing on cardio.

What you're trying to work off is fat, and the best way to do that is to eat right, and get in good solid cardio. Normally I'd advise at least thirty minutes of cardio four or five times a week. But since this was my shape-up week, my chance to really jump-start my fitness, I practically doubled that. I did an hour of cardio each day. I mostly get my cardio on the treadmill or in spin classes, and I try to mix it up with the stair-climber sometimes. Since this was my week to step it up, not only did I do cardio every day, I also did three days of circuit training. Talk about a kick in the @ss! It really wore me out, but it also made me feel great and accomplished. I made the most of my time off to get ahead of the game. I also focused on nutrition—every meal was superhealthy, and I avoided all the treats I occasionally allow myself. It's just one week—you can do anything for one week! The point of this is not to starve yourself (do not do that—it will only sabotage your long-term goals, not to mention interfere with your ability to take care of your baby) or exercise to the point of exhaustion. It's just a week to think about you.

You might not even see a difference on the scale by the end of the week, and that's fine. I guarantee there will be a difference in how you feel. And when you go back to your normal routine the following week you will get more out of your workouts, be more conscious of what you're eating, and have more energy. You'll also feel more in control of your health and a little less behind the eight ball, which is fantastic for your psyche.

I plan a week like this every now and then. After Megan was born I did it at two months, again at five months, and again at eight months. Every time it sharpens my focus, elevates my fitness level, and helps me feel so good. (I plan to keep doing it every so often, even when I'm not recovering from pregnancy!) As I write this, I'm starting a one-week "no crap" week. It's the first week of the new year, and it's my way of cleaning up my nutrition after the holidays. I'm consuming no sugar (no sugar substitutes either!), no alcohol, no meat, no preservatives, no dairy, and no caffeine for one week. I may be a little crabby at first, but I'm determined to see it through.

The key to making this happen is asking for help. You're a new mom—you can't do it alone and it is not too much to ask for. I have seen so many moms who have a "supermom" complex and want to prove that they can do it all. Believe me, I get it, but it's not realistic. No one expects you to do everything yourself, and you shouldn't even try. This is especially true during your shape-up week. No matter what your circumstances or schedule, when you pick this week, you should see it through. Explain your plan and your goals to your best friend, mom, *and* your husband. Get them on board to help you make it happen. And then GO FOR IT.

You don't need to leave town and hire full-time help for a week. But you do need someone else to take care of your baby, even for just one to two hours each day. You also need to carve out time to shop for and prepare healthy foods and, while the baby is sleeping or with someone else, to give yourself some pampering. Your husband will pitch in, and so can friends and relatives (you'll return the favor later). You might even pay a trusted babysitter to help you during one workout session.

Line up help in advance, plan your schedule for the entire week, and try to stick to it. Don't beat yourself up if you need to reschedule something, though. As I just said, you're a new mom—like you could forget that—and you're doing the best you can!

Shape-up Week Sample Menu

Here's what a day's worth of meals and snacks might look like this week. It's nothing too radical—just very healthy. (Remember, no sneaking treats—not this week.)

BREAKFAST: ½ cup high-fiber cereal, ½ cup low-fat Greek yogurt, and ½ cup berries

SNACK: Small handful of almonds

LUNCH: a 6-inch whole wheat pita with 3 ounces turkey, 1/8 avocado, lettuce, and tomato, and 1 piece of fruit

SNACK: carrot sticks or sliced jicama with tomato salsa

DINNER: 4 ounces grilled fish and mixed greens with chopped pears and dried cranberries tossed lightly with lemon juice and sea salt or light balsamic vinaigrette

Shape-up Week Sample Workout Schedule

MONDAY: 45-minute jog/walk and 30-minute training session with light weights

TUESDAY: 90-minute power yoga or Pilates session

WEDNESDAY: 60-minute cardio mix-up (20 minutes on stationary bike, 20 minutes on elliptical, 20 minutes on stair-climber) and 15-minute ab workout

THURSDAY: 60-minute spin class

FRIDAY: 60-minute treadmill workout (see page 164) and 30-minute training session with light weights

SATURDAY: 30-minute jog/walk *and* 30-minute stair-stepper plus 15-minute ab workout

SUNDAY: 60-minute spin class and 30-minute training session with light weights

NOTE: Each workout should be followed by at least 5 to 7 minutes of stretching!

MD MOVES: ✳ *60-Minute Serious Treadmill Workout*

I see people all the time next to me on the treadmill, mindlessly chugging away. They're off to a great start—they're getting their bodies moving, they're at the gym—but they aren't necessarily getting the most out of their time. Here's a more focused, more effective workout to try on the treadmill. It's a doozy: You will sweat and breathe hard and *feel it* when you do this one. (If this sounds like a little too much right now, try the 45-minute workout on page 145, and come back to this soon, when you're ready.)

0:00–1:30: Walk at 3.5 miles per hour, with the incline set at 2 percent. (All my trainers agree—no matter what you're doing on the treadmill—add a little incline if you want a more intense workout.)

1:30–3:00: Jog at 5.0 (keep incline at 2 percent).

3:00–4:00: Walk at 4.0 (same incline).

4:00–5:00: SPRINT. Which means RUN. As hard as you can. For ONE MINUTE. (Remember my "you can do anything for a week" motto? Well, it started as "you can do ANYTHING for one minute." It's true. You'll see.) Start off at 6.5 or 7.0.

5:00–6:00: Walk it out. (Keep the incline at 2 percent.) Catch your breath, 'cause you're about to sprint again.

6:00–7:00: Here you go again: RUN!!!

7:00–8:00: Bring it back to between 2.0 and 3.0, walk, breathe deeply, try to slow down your heart rate. Take a sip of water. Get ready . . .

8:00–9:00: Sprint it out! Give it everything you have. Run, run, run.

9:00–10:00: Awesome job. Walk it out. Catch your breath, and do a quick check on how your body handled that. If you're not new at this, and you're starting to recover quickly, maybe it's time to up the ante and try to run at a faster pace. Push yourself!

10:00–20:00: Raise the incline to 4 percent and set the pace between 4.5 and 5.5, get a good steady jog going, and maintain it. If you need to walk at any point, slow down. That's okay. The key is, the second you've recovered, push it back up to a jog. Get it going again! You have to challenge yourself.

20:00–25:00: Raise the incline to 6 and slow the treadmill WAY down to maybe .08 pace, and now do some lunges as you walk.

25:00–35:00: I know you're wearing out, so we're going to lower the incline to 1 percent (it's almost like going downhill) in time for more sprints. The slow lunges should have helped you get your heart rate back under control, so now it's time to elevate it again. Do a series of sprints, with 1 minute on and 1 minute to recover.

35:00–45:00: Oh man, I know, you're exhausted. I am too. Raise the incline to 15 percent. You read that right: all the way up. Set the pace between 3.0 and 3.5 and get your hands OFF THE TREADMILL. I put them on my hips or my head to remove temptation, and just climb that hill. One foot in front of the other, up, up, up.

45:00–50:00: Now for a little butt workout, slow the treadmill down to 1.8 to 2.4 (depending on your com-

continued on next page →

fort level) and turn around. I know it's weird, but I learned this in bootcamp classes years ago. You jog backward, and this time you can hold on to the treadmill bars until you get the hang of it.

50:00–57:00: Lower the incline to 1 percent and bring it back to the jog at 5.5 or as high as you can hang, with a good solid jog.

57:00–60:00: Good work! Now you gotta walk it out. Slow down to 4.0, then 3.0, then 2.0, each for 1 minute. Give yourself the time to relax and stretch out those legs. You did it!

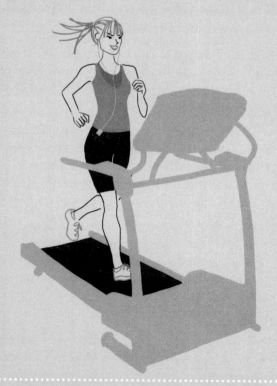

SHAPE-UP WEEK PAMPERING IDEAS

Even if it's something little, treat yourself to pampering every day.

1. Apply a moisturizing mask—to your hands! (They're probably dried out from all the hand-washing . . .)

2. Get a massage. (Lifting and carrying and bending over are tough on your muscles!)

3. Take a sauna or a steam, or soak in a tub with mois- turizing oils added.

4. Splurge on one great facial skin product (moistur- izer, serum, exfoliant, mask, eye cream) that you've been craving—and use it!

5. Get a haircut/color (I'm guessing you need it by now), don't skip the scalp massage, and say yes when they ask if you want them to blow out your hair. Who doesn't love a blow-out?

6. Give your hair a deep-conditioning treatment at home.

7. Buy a good book and enjoy it this week, even if you read for just twenty minutes before bed. Enjoy reading your favorite romance or chick lit novel, or mystery, or whatever helps you escape.

MD TUNES: ☀ *Shape-up Week Playlist*

When I'm having one of my shape-up weeks, I need good music to inspire me. These songs keep me going even when I feel like stopping. Find songs that you can lose yourself in. The tough parts of the workout will go by faster, and you'll find yourself using the music to push you. To me, music is the key to a good workout. Try this playlist when you really want to keep moving!

"Hurts So Good" by John Mellencamp

"Right Now" by Van Halen

"I'm Yours" by Jason Mraz

"Beautiful" by Christina Aguilera

"Your Body Is a Wonderland" by John Mayer

"Man in the Mirror" by Michael Jackson

"Authority Song" by John Mellencamp

"I'm a Believer" by Smash Mouth

"Every Little Thing She Does Is Magic" by The Police

"Don't Stop Believin'" by Journey

"Can't Hold Us Down" (feat. Lil' Kim) by Christina Aguilera

"One" by U2

"Wonderful Tonight" by Eric Clapton

Months Six
Through Nine

If you've been following the plan in *The Mommy Diet,* by now I'm guessing you're seeing some real, tangible progress in terms of how your body looks and feels. Nice! One of the moments that lets you know you're really getting there is the first time you're able to fit into the same-size clothes you wore before you even thought about getting pregnant. For me, when it finally happened, I was especially excited about fitting into my prepregnancy jeans. It's such a great feeling. All that hard work and sweat *does* eventually pay off.

When I fit into size twenty-sevens after about seven months—no, it did not happen sooner than that—I freaked out (in a good way.) Having struggled with body image and my weight my whole life, fitting into a twenty-seven True Religion jean made me feel really good, and proud of myself. My body didn't look quite like it did before pregnancy, though. If anything, with all the work I was doing, it was better! That's not to say I was stick thin—for one thing, I noticed my butt was changing shape. Corina, my makeup artist and friend, told me I was developing a "J-Lo" butt. (You know, a bubble-shaped backside.) I was a little hesitant to embrace it at first, but the more I worked out, the more I saw what she was talking about, and I liked it.

I also started to notice that my clavicle was more defined. Take a look in the mirror and see if you notice the same thing. Don't your neck and jawline look sharper? That's because you've been shedding a layer of fat! Calling attention to these body parts is a great way to remind you of how far you've come. If you're anything like me, you may still be frustrated about certain parts of your body (for me it's thighs, stomach, and arms), but don't just think about those—check out the body parts that look amazing and show your progress. Take a second to be proud of what you've accomplished so far, rather than always dwelling on how far you have to go.

Fitness

By now you've established a good base fitness level. You're strong, you've got endurance, and you feel good. (If you're new to this book and just getting started now, back up a few chapters and follow the fitness plans in order. Begin slowly and steadily, building up your strength and cardiovascular fitness.)

Guess what? It's time to kick it up a notch.

Not every workout should feel like a walk in the park. Sometimes you need to leave it all at the gym, and come away totally sweaty and spent. This can be exhilarating, as long as you are healthy and in good enough shape to go all out.

So yes, the workouts get harder, but the results are really worth it. My coauthor, Christie, started training for the New York City Marathon six months after her baby was born, and she ran it when her baby was eight months old. During that time she says the extra cardio work (lots of running!) was the tipping point, and by race day she was feeling amazing, and easily fitting into her skinny jeans. (Okay, she didn't feel so amazing at mile twenty, but that's another story.) Also, as a side note, she was still breastfeeding throughout all of this. She actually brought an inexpensive manual breast pump to the starting line so she could "pump and dump" right before race time, and though she got some really strange looks, she did it—no joke—while the national anthem was playing. So for those of you using breastfeeding as an excuse . . . yup, you can't use it anymore. You don't need to train for a marathon to get these results, either. It just takes a little more intensity, and you're there. You can do it!

1. Get into the habit of consistently working out four or five days per week. That might sound daunting, but it's so good for you—and if you make it a priority and focus on it for a few weeks, it will become a habit. Of course, I know you won't be able to work out for an hour or two on each of those days, and that's okay. Even thirty or forty-five minutes, if you do it regularly, can give you amazing results. Aim for at least twenty minutes, though. Some experts think you don't really get to the good calorie and fat burning till after twenty minutes of cardio.

Think about your week and when you can fit in these workouts. Can you work out on both weekend days? Can you do one early-morning workout before the baby gets up? Can you go to the gym at lunchtime? Can you take a yoga class one evening? Can you trade babysitting with a friend so you can take a spin class one afternoon? Map out your schedule and make a realistic plan. Also, if you find yourself with unexpected free time (I know, I know . . . yeah, right!), throw in an extra workout for good measure.

As I've said before, I work out every day that I can. This means some weeks I work out every single day, and some weeks I get to work out only two or three times. But most weeks I manage to get four or five workouts, and I feel so much better when I do.

2. Go for a morning workout when you can. If you have the luxury of time, several experts have told me that the ideal time to work out is in the morning. When you work out first thing in the morning (after a light breakfast), your metabolism is elevated for the whole day, helping you burn calories more efficiently all day long. Plus, when you've worked out in the morning, it's *done*—nothing is going to make you miss your workout that day. A morning workout certainly isn't something I can do all the time, but I try to do it when I have the time. I often squeeze it in before my kids are even awake. Keep this in the back of your mind for weekends, or whenever you happen to have the choice.

3. Add interval training to your routine. This is the best thing ever for busy moms, because you can complete a really effective workout in thirty minutes, and Elise Gulan says it's the most effective way to lose fat and get toned. She explains that high-intensity interval training (HIIT) involves a warm-up period (five to ten minutes), six to ten repetitions of high-intensity cardio exercise alternating with medium-intensity cardio exercise (say, thirty seconds of sprinting, one minute of jogging, thirty seconds of sprinting, another one minute of jogging, and so on for at least six cycles), and then a cool-down period of five to ten minutes.

The key with this kind of exercise is that you make the high-intensity segments truly intense. Go all out! Running isn't the only option for HIIT. Elise suggests interval spin classes, interval cardio-strength classes, or doing it on your own at the gym on the elliptical, treadmill, or bike. Warm up for several minutes, then go full force for up to one minute, recover for twice as long as you sprinted, and then keep repeating the cycle, at least six times. As you do more interval training, you'll get stronger and fitter and be able to "go hard" longer. Try to make at least one of your workouts each week a HIIT workout.

4. Continue to balance your cardio work with strength training. Elise explains that building lean muscle mass boosts your resting metabolic rate, meaning you scorch more calories all day long, even at rest. This doesn't mean bulking up with heavy weights. Elise says yoga is one of the best means of strengthening, because it also stretches you and has a mind-body element that's so good for you. Do at least one or two workouts per week that are really focused on strengthening (a yoga or Pilates class or DVD; another strength-and-tone class

MD MOVES: ✷ *Sample Week of Workouts*

MONDAY: Day off (but try to take a walk with your baby or walk to do errands or walk to work!)

TUESDAY: 30 minutes of HIIT

WEDNESDAY: 60-minute mind-body strengthening class (such as yoga, Pilates, or Bar Method)

THURSDAY: 45 minutes on elliptical trainer, Nordic ski machine, or stair-climber (or a mix of all three) or jog or take a kickboxing class, plus 15-minute abs-and-arms workout

FRIDAY: Day off (but again, try to walk as much as you can, and you're still stretching at night, right?)

SATURDAY: 60-minute spin class, plus 15 minutes of strength training with light weights

SUNDAY: 90-minute yoga class or DVD, plus hike with the family or 30 minutes of cardio (jog, stationary bike, elliptical trainer)

or DVD, such as Core Fusion, Bar Method, Lotte Berk, or Physique 57; a circuit class; or even rock climbing) and then incorporate some strength training (ab work, training with light weights and your own body weight) on one or two other workout days, too.

5. Sample other intense workouts you've been considering. Have you ever tried boxing or kickboxing? It's incredible—a

tough and exhausting workout when it's done right, and yet so much fun, not to mention a great stress reliever. The time flies by. Or take a really challenging hike. There's a state park in my neighborhood that I visit for outdoor workouts when I can. I just recently discovered a hike that takes me up the steep side of a mountain, and there are parts where I'm practically rock climbing. It's invigorating. I love that my heart is pounding, and I'm more focused on my next foothold than the fact that I'm working out.

MD TUNES: ✳ *Interval Training Playlist*

This mix alternates between fast songs and slow songs, so you can always have the right beat going for the all-out moments and the recovery period.

"Tainted Love" (7" Single) by Soft Cell

"Blister in the Sun" by Violent Femmes

"Thank You" by Alanis Morissette

"Bad Moon Rising" by Creedence Clearwater Revival

"Girls" by Beastie Boys

"Take Me Away" by Plain White T's

"I Wanna Be Sedated" by The Ramones

"One" by Mary J. Blige (feat. U2)

"Laid" by Better Than Ezra

"Lost!" by Coldplay

"Hard to Handle" (Live) by The Black Crowes

"You Give Love a Bad Name" by Bon Jovi

"Lose Yourself" by Eminem

"No One" by Alicia Keys

"Should I Stay or Should I Go" by The Clash

"Just Breathe" by Pearl Jam

Food

By now healthfully eating should be an ingrained habit. Sure, you may indulge in a treat from time to time—and that's not only acceptable but a good idea—but for the most part you're eating lots of veggies and fruits, getting plenty of calcium and iron and other vitamins and minerals, and sticking to lean meats and fish, while avoiding meals that are superheavy, deep-fried, or filled with saturated fats.

1. Eat 25 to 30 grams of fiber per day, increasing your fiber intake gradually if you're not close to that level now. I have some exciting news. You've stuck with me for this long, so now you get to hear it. There is a secret weapon that you can use for weight loss and maintenance. As Meg Moreta says, if there's a magic bullet, fiber is it. Getting the right amount of fiber is not only very healthy for your heart and your intestines, it's a trick that can help you stay trim forever, because it helps you feel full longer—and because part of the food isn't broken down, so you never absorb the calories. Woohoo!

A few things to know: This does not mean you should eat twice as much fiber as you need. That will just clog up your insides and make you feel nasty. Stick with the recommended amount—it's likely more than you're getting now, because you really have to be conscious about it to eat that much fiber. Meg explains that the average American gets only 10 to 12 grams of fiber per day. The best sources of fiber are whole grains, beans, fruits, and vegetables. Here are some of my favorite fiber sources:

High-fiber cereal, like Raisin Bran (about 8 grams per serving)

Raspberries (8 grams per cup)

Pears (5 grams per medium pear with skin)

Ground flaxseed (about 3 grams per tablespoon)—mix it into a shake or sprinkle it on your cereal

Black beans (about 8 grams per ½ cup cooked beans)

Artichoke hearts (about 5 grams per 4 to 5 hearts)

Spinach (about 4 grams per cup of fresh raw spinach)

High-fiber whole wheat tortilla (about 7 grams of fiber)

Almonds (about 3 grams per ounce)

Avocados (about 2 grams of fiber per 2 tablespoons)

Tip: Check the label of any cereal you're thinking about buying at the grocery store. If it doesn't have at least 3 grams of fiber per serving, pick another one!

So a day when you eat about 30 grams of fiber might look like this:

Breakfast: Greek yogurt with ½ cup fresh raspberries

Snack: medium pear

Lunch: high-fiber tortilla with ½ cup black beans, low-fat cheese, and 2 tablespoons avocado

Snack: handful of almonds

Dinner: grilled chicken or fish with spinach salad

MD EATS: ✳ *Easy, Healthy Chicken Dishes*

Skinless chicken breasts are a great source of lean protein, and they are so versatile. Here's how I prepare chicken, with several ideas for variations—and you can do all of these with just one pan. When you're in the mood for chicken and you want to cook something quick, healthy, and tasty, give one of these a try.

But first, a few things to keep in mind for cooking chicken: Take the time to preheat the skillet as directed by recipes. I know you're in a hurry, but this is important if you want the chicken to cook evenly and thoroughly. Also, people usually err on the side of overcooking chicken because they don't want it raw. If you cook chicken enough, you will get the hang of it—you don't want it pink and raw, but please strive for a still-moist chicken breast. Finally, look for organic, free-range chicken whenever possible. Okay, here are my go-to chicken recipes:

ONION AND FENNEL CHICKEN (serves 4): Season 4 small chicken breasts with 1 teaspoon Basic Chicken Rub (see page 180) and 1 teaspoon fennel seeds. Preheat a skillet over medium heat for 2 minutes. Spray the skillet lightly with Pam or cooking oil (I put oil in a pump canister from Sur La Table). Add the seasoned chicken to the pan and cook for about 3 minutes on each side. Remove the chicken from the skillet and set it aside. Add 1 tablespoon extra-virgin olive oil to the skillet. Add 1 fennel bulb (chopped), 1 large white onion (chopped), and 2 garlic cloves (chopped); sauté until softened (the onion should be translucent), about 10 minutes. Add ½ cup dry white wine or chicken stock and let cook, scraping the sides of the pan occasionally, until the sauce has thickened slightly. Then add

→

3/4 cup chicken stock and 3/4 cup water and whisk together. Return the chicken to the pan, cover, and bring the liquid to a gentle boil. After that point, let the liquid reduce by half, about 5 minutes. Serve the chicken with its sauce and a green vegetable, like broccoli or green beans, or a mixed green salad with some fennel added to tie the flavors together.

TAHINI CHICKEN (serves 4): In a small bowl, combine 1 tablespoon onion powder, 2 teaspoons dried oregano, 1 tablespoon grated lemon peel, 1 tablespoon salt, 1 teaspoon pepper, 1/3 cup sesame tahini, and 1/4 cup sesame seeds. Cut 4 small chicken breasts into 1-inch cubes and use the spice mixture to season the chicken. Preheat a skillet over medium heat, spray lightly with cooking oil, and cook the chicken cubes for 3 minutes on each side. Serve with brown rice or whole wheat couscous, about ½ cup per person.

CHICKEN WITH DRIED CHERRIES (serves 4): Cut 4 small chicken breasts into 1-inch cubes. In a medium bowl, combine 2 tablespoons flour, 1 tablespoon curry powder (mild, unless you dig some major spice), and 1 teaspoon salt. Toss the chicken pieces in the curry flour and brush off the excess. Preheat a skillet over medium heat. Spray the pan lightly with cooking oil and cook the chicken for about 2 minutes per side, to brown it for flavor (you will cook it more in the liquid). Remove the chicken from the skillet and set it aside. Add about 1 tablespoon olive oil to the skillet. Add 1 small white onion (chopped) and 2 stalks celery (chopped) and cook for 3 to 5 minutes over medium heat. Return the cooked chicken to the skillet and stir. Add ¼ cup dried cherries and ¼ cup water, and bring the water to a boil.

continued on next page →

Turn the heat down to medium-low and let simmer for about 3 minutes. Stir in 1/3 cup light coconut milk. Serve with whole wheat couscous or brown rice (about ½ cup per person), or use as a chicken salad (using only a spare amount of sauce in this case).

CHICKEN AND CABBAGE (serves 4): In a small bowl, combine 1 teaspoon caraway seeds, ¼ teaspoon allspice, 1 teaspoon salt, and 1 teaspoon pepper. Use the spice blend to season 4 small chicken breasts. Preheat a skillet over medium heat and spray lightly with cooking oil. Cook the chicken breasts for 3 minutes on each side and set aside. For the sauce, use the same skillet and add 1 tablespoon olive oil to the hot pan. Sauté 2 shallots (chopped) for 2 minutes, then add 3 cups shredded red cabbage, 1/2 cup chicken stock, 2 tablespoons vinegar, and 1 teaspoon brown sugar; turn the heat up to medium-high and cook, stirring, until the cabbage is coated with glaze. After about 2 minutes, return the cooked chicken to the skillet and cook for about 6 more minutes. Garnish with chopped chives.

BASIC CHICKEN RUB: I have some of this on hand all the time to season chicken before I grill it or prepare it in some other way. Use it to season chicken breasts lightly on both sides. Be sure to clean your hands carefully before doing anything else after you season raw chicken! To make it, combine 2 tablespoons dried basil, 2 tablespoons dried oregano, 2 tablespoons onion powder, 2 tablespoons garlic powder, 2 tablespoons ground pepper, 2 tablespoons salt, and 2 tablespoons sweet paprika and mix well.

If you haven't been getting your recommended daily dose of fiber, increase your intake gradually so your system gets used to it. And then try to get enough fiber every day.

2. Drink plenty of water! Are you getting sick of me saying that yet? It's so important, and it's not hard to do, but it's easy to *forget* to do, especially when you're a busy mom. If you're eating a high-fiber diet, getting water is really key—without it you could feel constipated or gassy. These are not things a hot mama wants to feel! Drink eight to ten glasses a day, or fill a re-usable water bottle and commit to finishing it however many times per day will give you sixty-four ounces or more.

Megan is always reminding me to drink more water. I know that sounds weird, but seriously, my one-year-old daughter loves to drink water, and it's such a good reminder. Before you get old enough to prefer soda or wine or whatever, you just love drinking good old-fashioned water.

3. Have guilt-free treats on hand. Sure, you should indulge in a bite or two of something decadent from time to time, but many of us get cravings for, say, a taste of something sweet fairly often. I allow my kids more dessert treats than I allow myself. But Ben hates to eat his alone. He always asks me to sit with him while he's enjoying a homemade popsicle or an oc-casional ice cream, because he is required to eat them at the kitchen table. (I am not cleaning that off the walls all over the house!) Sitting there watching him enjoy a yummy treat can be torture when I'm trying to be good, so I came up with a few treats I could enjoy sans guilt:

* Frozen fruit: It's nothing fancy, but it's somehow more of a treat than regular fruit. I can't explain why. Frozen grapes or a frozen banana (maybe with a little dark chocolate sprinkled over it) can be fabulous.

* Frozen Greek yogurt: You know the Greek yogurt I recommend all the time? You can throw that in the freezer, too. Cut up some strawberries or blueberries or whatever fruit you like, mix them in, and dig into a healthy version of yummy frozen yogurt.

* Grilled fruit: Dave had the ingenious idea of throwing a few peaches on the grill one night last summer. I added some cinnamon and a drizzle of honey just before serving, and that's become a new family favorite. Try peaches and plums and nectarines when they are in season, or try pineapple and orange slices—experiment with your favorites!

* Dried figs: They're like a Fig Newton without the bready cookie. They're fairly high in calories, though, so just have two or three.

4. Add flavor to food with herbs and spices. Cooking at home is a good way to know exactly what you're eating and to make sure it's healthy. If you want to make food that's loaded with flavor, but not with fat, use lots of herbs and spices. Rocco DiSpirito gave me great tips on how to work with herbs and spices in my kitchen. First, he notes that you need to replace

MD EATS: ❋ *Spice It Up!*

Here are a few of chef Rocco DiSpirito's ideas for using herbs and spices every day:

Chili powder for soups and stews

Curry powder for soups, stews, and (of course) curries

Cinnamon for soups and apple pie

Cumin for anything Mexican or Middle Eastern

Crushed red pepper flakes for everything, especially pasta

Dried oregano and dried tarragon for flavored vinegars and vinaigrettes and dry rubs for meat and fish

Dried rosemary for steaks and lamb

Fresh basil for salads and pasta

Fresh cilantro for avocados and tuna dishes

Fresh Italian flat-leaf parsley for everything

your dried herbs and spices if they've been sitting around too long losing flavor. As he says, if you still have a jar of spice that you had in college, or you've packed your spices and moved with them more than once, it's time to get new ones. He explains that age and neglect are the enemies of dried herbs and spices. He also encourages experimentation—buy fresh and dried herbs and spices in small quantities, and play around; use them every day. See the Spice It Up! box above for some of his favorite ways to incorporate spices into everyday foods.

Fashion

Hey there, pretty lady, how you doin'? You're looking *good* these days. Don't fret if you aren't quite in the shape you ultimately want to be in. Believe me, if you're sticking to the plan in this book, you will get there—and you look amazing already. So if someone says, "Wow, I can't believe you just had a baby—you look great!" you need to accept the compliment and say, "Thank you!"

I am guessing the few items you acquired to get you through the postbaby transition period aren't fitting so well anymore. I went through a phase when I had to switch to a smaller pair of jeans every other week. It feels good! As you get fitter and slimmer, be aware that some women's sizes change permanently after pregnancy. Not just shoe size, either. Some women find that their rib cages are forever a bra size bigger after hosting a whole other person inside of them. Also, your hips loosen and rotate outward during pregnancy, and it's common to have your hip bones just a little wider spread than before. Sorry, it's part of the deal. One smile from your child, and it's all worth it. I'm just telling you in case certain slim skirts or favorite bras seem extremely snug even after all your hard work. This could be a factor. Don't get upset—it's just part of nature. Find what looks good on you and fits now.

1. Reassess how things are fitting you once a month (or more often, as needed). If the one-size-up pieces you had postbaby don't look so good, stop wearing them. Put them away if you think you might get pregnant again, or pass them along

to a friend in the same boat. Venture back into your prebaby wardrobe and try on everything. Nope, not everything will fit. I'll tell you that right now. No biggie. But some things surely will—and as you get fitter and fitter, even more things will fit you. It's fun to rediscover all those old favorites that you haven't been able to wear for a while! (When you're doing this, remember that if something theoretically fits but you just don't like it or think it looks good on you, give it away.)

2. Around month eight or nine, find a hot pair of superstylish jeans that fit you beautifully. I adore jeans. They are perfect so much of the time. I wear them on TV a lot, they are sexy for date nights, and they are good for crawling around on the floor with your baby, too. I think it's hard to have too many pairs of jeans that make you look and feel great. I'm not talking about "mom jeans" (you know what I mean)—go for some sweet designer denim. You can find fabulous jeans at every price point. Get them hemmed to a nice heel length. If you can afford it, get another pair that you hem for flats, too. But if you do only one pair, go for the dressy heel/boot length that you can roll up twice for flats if you want.

3. Under your jeans, or whatever else you're wearing, you need some great underwear. Even if no one else sees what kind of skivvies you've got going on (and you never know when someone might!), you're aware of them. You're going to feel just a little more confident and a little more together if they are good-looking. Do you really feel like a hot mom in worn-out, stained, drooping panties? Plus, there's the issue of panty lines.

My stylist, Liza Whitcraft, is a huge fan of thongs. Comfortable thongs, that is. My favorites are Hanky Panky (so comfy), and Liza also suggests Cosabella's cotton-blend thongs. Lots of companies do inexpensive knock-offs of these now, too. If you're not a fan of the thong fit, I get it—they take some getting used to. You don't always need them for jeans; they're more for slacks, fitted dresses, and Juicy sweats. Always keep an eye out for that panty line when you're looking in the mirror. If you see one, something's wrong!

4. Beware the "muffin top." If you wear jeans or pants that are too tight, they can push a layer of flesh up over the top edge so it spills out—kind of like the top of an oversized muffin. It might look enticing on a baked good (not that you're eating oversized muffins, right?) but it doesn't look good on you. If anything you try on gives you muffin top, it doesn't fit. Don't wear it.

5. Also keep an eye out for back fat. Sometimes a bra that doesn't fit right can grab and pinch you across your back, especially right behind your underarm. It's not just you—even superskinny actresses I know get this. When you're trying on tight-fitting shirts, now that you look so fabulous from head-on, don't forget to turn around and check to see how it looks from the back. If it doesn't look right, there are great bras that can smooth you out. Spanx (the makers of the best undergarment accessories since hose were invented) makes an amazing bra that's supportive without creating unattractive dents in your back.

6. Speaking of bras, when you're no longer breastfeeding, go to a good lingerie store to get measured to find out your true bra size. You don't need to buy all your bras there, but make sure you know your size, because it may have changed completely, and wearing a bra that fits can make the difference between clothes looking just okay or looking fantastic. There's the expanded rib cage factor, and many women lose a cup size after they stop breastfeeding. Was I the only one who didn't know that was going to happen? So not fair. Still, it's better to know the truth and deal with it.

Self-Care

You've been doing the mom thing for months now. It's a good time to take stock of how much attention you're paying to you! I've mentioned many times how important it is to take care of yourself, for your own good and for the good of your entire family. So, let's check in: Are you doing it? Are you really doing it? Here are some rules to follow to make sure you're doing it. No cheating.

1. Pick one small thing that you want to do every day (apart from exercising and eating well—though, of course, you should keep that up!) because it makes you feel good. Reading an entertaining book for twenty minutes before bed. Writing in a journal. Lighting candles, lying on the couch, and listening to your favorite music. Using a gentle exfoliating scrub on

your arms and legs in the shower so your skin is supersoft. Whatever your favorite little ritual is, make it a true ritual. Do it every day!

2. Okay, now pick one slightly bigger thing that you want to do once a week because it makes you feel good. Meeting a girlfriend for a glass of wine. Visiting an art museum. Walking on the beach. Getting a manicure (following the tips for a healthy manicure on page 13, of course). Make it a ritual and do it every week!

3. You probably know where I'm going here: Pick one big treat—it can be a bit of a splurge, or it doesn't have to cost a thing—and do it once a month. Every month! Don't just do it for one month and then let it slip away. You can mix this up a bit if there are several different bigger treats you crave, but be sure to pick things that make you feel amazing. Maybe a hot stone massage (ooooh), or a day trip to your favorite destination (a nature preserve or a seaside town), a sleepover with your girlfriends (you're not too old for that—bring on the chick flicks, the wine, and lots of laughing), a night at a hotel just for you, an evening at your favorite indie movie house . . . whatever makes you totally relaxed or happy or blissful.

Romance

Keeping your relationship hot after having a baby isn't easy, and it doesn't get a whole lot easier even once those first few months of sleepless nights are over, and you're back to feeling more like yourself mentally and physically. Things have changed. It's not just the two of you any longer. You have more responsibilities and much less time for yourselves (individually and as a couple). And this is how it's going to be for the next, oh, eighteen years. Please don't put your relationship on the back burner till then! Because having a healthy, loving relationship with your spouse is one of the best things you can do, for each other and for your kids. It's so worth it to work at it, every day.

Of course, as your kids get older and maybe you have another child, things keep changing. There's nothing quite like having your toddler walk in while you and your hubby are getting intimate. Even if he just calls out "Mommy? I need a drink of water!" it can be a total buzz-kill to the mood. Dave and I both agreed on a no-kids-in-our-bed policy to maintain our privacy and relationship space, but each couple makes their own choice about what's best for their family. If you share a family bed, or have your infant in your bedroom just for convenience, you have to work even harder to allow for couple time. (And in particular to allow for spontaneity.) However you decide to go about it, just give it the attention and effort your relationship deserves. You can thank me later.

Here are a few things—they're not always easy—to think about trying in your relationship.

1. Say you're sorry. Feeling overwhelmed and tired, worrying about a child who is sick or fussy, wondering when you'll ever have enough time to get everything done . . . it can all make

you pretty irritable. And that's when you might snap at your partner, or blame him for something that's not his fault, or just be cranky with him. Watch out for this, and when you do it— we all do!—apologize right away. Be sincere, explain what's really going on, and try not to do it again anytime soon.

2. If you need something, tell your partner, and be as specific and straightforward as possible. As the mom, you shoulder so much responsibility. It's easy to try to do it all . . . and then feel resentful because your partner isn't helping. But I'm betting he wants to help more. He just doesn't know what to do! I mentioned earlier in the book how important it is to ask for help while you're pregnant, because you physically can't do everything. Now, technically, you probably can—but that doesn't mean you should.

Ask him to empty the diaper pail or vacuum the playroom or clean the baby's bottles. I'm telling you, he'll be psyched to know there's a concrete way that he can really help you. Ask for time, too—for you to work out or get a massage or have dinner with a friend. I'm hoping you've been doing this all along, but I want to remind you to keep doing it! Keeping any resentment out of your relationship will go a long way to making you both a lot happier, and happy to be with each other.

3. Don't get so wrapped up in your baby that you ignore your partner. You might think this could never happen, but it does. There are days when I get home from a long day of work or an overnight trip and I'm so excited to see the kids that I basically forget Dave's there and go straight to Ben and Megan (which I

know I shouldn't do—because I don't like it when Dave does that to me!). Yes, you're in love with your baby, but you have time to give your spouse a hug and a kiss when you get home, or have a conversation with him while the baby's around. Find ways to connect as you enjoy your baby together.

4. Once you've asked for help from your partner, or when he's in charge while you hit the gym or go out with your friends, don't tell him how to parent. I mean, you should give him the highlights before you go (when the next bottle is due; what time to put the baby down for a nap), but beyond that, you have to learn to let that go. He might not burp the baby the same way you do, or follow your precise technique for diaper changes. That's fine; in fact, it's healthy for the baby to get used to a little variety.

Many marriages hit rocky points because the mom wants everything done her way, and that's just not fair to your husband or the baby. Your husband is bonding the best way he can, and inevitably he's going to do it his way anyway, so keep your cringing to a minimum, and just walk away if you can't watch him changing the diaper. He'll figure it out and be a more confident dad if he isn't always worried, waiting for a critique from you.

5. Have sex regularly. (No, you don't have to do it every night. Try for once a week, or a schedule that seems right for you.) I know you don't feel like it a lot of the time. I get it. I'm sure some readers (and critics!) aren't going to like this, but I think sometimes you need to give it a try even when you think you

don't want to. But don't be a martyr about it. If you're going to do it even though you're not totally into it in the moment, don't make a big point of explaining that you're not in the mood! He doesn't want pity sex from you. Well, he'd probably take it at this point, but that's not your goal, is it? It doesn't have to take a long time; it doesn't have to keep you up for an extra three hours. A quickie will be perfectly (or mostly) satisfying for him, and I'm guessing you're going to feel better afterward, too—more like the sexy woman you are, and definitely more connected to your partner. So if he makes a move on you and you're not in the mood, don't always shove him away. Give it a try for a few minutes to see if you get into it. (If you don't, tell him what's going on, of course.) And one other thing: You should initiate sex sometimes, too!

Note: You may not want to know this, but I've read that sex actually cures headaches. Kind of makes that cliché "I have a headache" excuse moot, right? I'm just pointing out that even if you don't want to have sex in the moment he initiates, don't necessarily say no right away . . . give your body a second to adjust and open to the idea. You may change your mind if you give yourself the chance.

6. Remember the massage I already suggested that you should treat yourself to? Try trading massages with your lover. It's free and it feels great. You both can do it the same night, or one night at a time, and then allow things to follow their natural course. Make sure you start off by getting a really deep, thorough massage . . . and then do the same for him when it's his turn.

Kick Start!

Maybe you've gone nine months since your baby was born without paying much attention to your diet or exercise regimen. Maybe you've even gone nine years since your baby was born without taking good care of yourself. Or maybe you've tried here and there, but the pounds aren't budging and you're not feeling so hot. Whatever the reason, if you need to kick-start your health and well-being in a big way, this is the chapter for you. Commit to following this program for one to six months (or as long as you need), and then check out the plan in the Mommy Maintenance chapter beginning on page 213.

There are just two rules to keep in mind before we begin: First, do not give yourself a hard time or beat yourself up for being where you are today. That does no good. You are where you are, and now you're thinking about getting healthy. You rock! Let's start moving forward. Second, do not give this a half-assed effort and then give up. You've got to be all in. You've got to do this! No excuses, no laziness, no trying here and there. This is your time to get healthy. You can make it happen. Yes, you can. You're about to commit to adopting many amazing habits that will change your life for the better. Let's GO!

Tip: If you're using this kick-start plan to go from a not-so-healthy lifestyle to a healthy one, all the changes can seem overwhelming—it's a lot to remember. So give yourself a cheat sheet. Make a quick checklist of the things you need to do every day (see alisonsweeney.com for our version of the checklist), and refer to it often.

Another tip: Talk to your partner about the changes you are making, and get him on board to support you as you adopt a healthier lifestyle. Not only will you need his help with childcare, but it's good to educate him a little along the way so he knows what a healthy meal looks like (and doesn't inadvertently sabotage your efforts by making a huge pasta dinner with creamy sauce to help you "carbo load" or something) and understands why you need regular workout time. Guys can be obtuse sometimes—so don't be afraid to spell things out for him. Maybe he'll be inspired to get fitter along with you!

Fitness

It's so easy to let fitness get away from you. You're busy, you don't have much (make that any) spare time, and if you're not careful, exercise can fall to the very bottom of your to-do list. I understand how that happens, but I also know that something has to change. If lack of time is your reason (read: excuse) for not working out, next time you sit and watch an hour of

TV, consider that you could have had a great workout in the same amount of time. Exercise is so, so, so important for your health, and for your self-esteem. Especially if you've been fairly sedentary for a while (like, you can't exactly remember the last time you had a workout, but you're pretty sure it wasn't during this presidential administration), please check with your doctor to make sure it's okay to start a regular fitness regime, and see if anything's off-limits. Once you have the go-ahead, it's time to get moving!

1. Commit to being active every day. Every. Single. Day. More specifically, commit to getting at least thirty minutes of concentrated cardiovascular activity (walking, riding a bike, hiking, swimming, playing a sport, using the elliptical trainer) five days per week.

2. Commit to doing some form of strength training every other day. Strength training helps you get stronger (right, obviously), look great (hello, sculpted muscles), and burn more calories all day long (muscles burn more than fat). Try yoga or Pilates class, abs classes, circuit classes, or your own at-home routine. Here's a simple ten- to fifteen-minute routine to try—between reps of each exercise, be doing another exercise so you never stop moving, and you finish quickly!

Strength Moves

* Plank pose (see page 117)

* Lunges (see page 71)

* Jumping jacks (do them for two minutes straight and get your heart rate up)

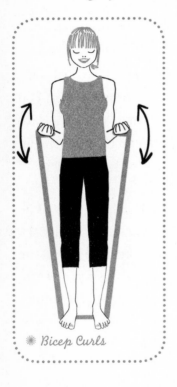

* Bicep Curls

* Biceps curls: Stand on the center of a resistance band with your feet shoulder width apart. Hold one end of the band in each hand with your palms facing up and your elbows close to your sides. Keeping your elbows pressed into your rib cage, slowly curl your hands toward your shoulders, keeping your wrists straight. Lower slowly, resisting momentum on the way down, and repeat.

* Ab curls (see page 117)

* "Burpees" (That's what we call these at my gym): Drop down, do one push-up, hop your feet up next to your hands, then push off with your feet and jump into the air as high as you can. When

you land, immediately put your hands down near your feet, and jump back into a push-up position. Repeat! Build up to being able to do twenty reps.

* Triceps dips (see page 92) or triceps extensions (see page 44)

* Bicycle crunches: Lie flat on the floor with your lower back pressed into the ground. Place your hands gently behind your head (don't use them to pull your head up) with your elbows pointing to the side, and use your abdominal muscles to pull your head, neck, and upper back off the floor. Bend your knees at a 90-degree angle, with your shins parallel to the floor. Using *only* your abdominal muscles, move your left elbow toward your right knee (which should remain at a 90-degree angle) while extending your left leg straight but keeping it off the ground. With control, simultaneously bend your left knee to 90 degrees, extend

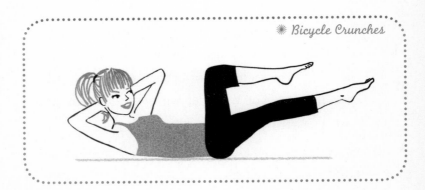

* Bicycle Crunches

your right leg, and move your right elbow toward your left knee. This is one repetition. Build up to three sets of ten repetitions.

* Jump lunges: Get into a lunge pose—see page 71—and sink into it! Then leap into the air, switching legs, and landing in a lunge on the other side. Build up to fifty reps.

* Shoulder presses (see page 44. You can be seated for this.)

* Jabs: Holding very light weights, make a punching motion with your right arm for fifteen reps, then do it with your left arm for fifteen reps, then for thirty seconds, punch as fast as you can going back and forth with both arms.

* Single-leg standups (see page 91)

3. In addition to your focused workouts, take each and every opportunity to add movement to your day. Here are a few ways to do that:

* To go up or down a few floors, take the stairs. Do you really need an escalator or elevator to get from the first to the second floor of the mall? Come on. (Yes, if you've got a stroller with you, it's okay to take the elevator!)

* Don't use the closest parking space. Park a little farther away and walk a few extra feet.

MD MOVES: ✳ *The Injury Excuse*

Lots of people get unhealthy or obese and use an injury as an excuse for not getting fit. I'm not saying an injury isn't a major restriction and impediment. It is, definitely. Being unable to complete a full workout can make getting into shape extremely difficult, and I certainly don't have the knowledge or expertise to tell you specifically what you should be doing for your injuries. But I do want to share a few thoughts on this subject. First of all, when it comes to getting in shape, the relative importance of diet and exercise isn't fifty-fifty. I think it's more like seventy-thirty. So if you're unable to work out, you have even *more* reason to eat well, because you aren't able to burn as many calories as you could if you worked out. So focus on your nutrition as much as possible. Second, if only one part of your body is injured, there's still the rest of you. Contestants on *The Biggest Loser* have proven that you can work around an injury by being EXTREMELY CAREFUL, and by focusing on other body parts. Don't let an injury stop you completely if it doesn't have to. I've seen girls in arm casts doing cardio on the elliptical at my gym, people with knee injuries on the stationary bikes, people with back problems swimming. I don't know your issues, so I'm not telling you exactly what to do, but my point is that you can work around many injuries; you just have to make it a priority to figure out how. If you have an injury, you're probably dealing with a doctor of some kind. Get him or her on board to help you figure out what you *can* do! And then *do it*!

* When you're running errands, see if you can walk between a few of them instead of driving everywhere.

* If you take public transportation, hop off one stop early and walk the rest of the way.

* Think of housecleaning, yardwork, and other chores as a way to burn calories—and do them vigorously. Yeah! Your house will look great, as a bonus.

MD TUNES: * *Kick-Start Playlist*

Need to get motivated? Here's a great hour-long playlist.

"Get the Party Started" by P!nk

"No Sleep Till Brooklyn" by Beastie Boys

"Single Ladies (Put a Ring On It)" by Beyoncé

"Boom Boom Pow" by Black Eyed Peas

"Dirrty" (feat. Redman) by Christina Aguilera

"Music" by Madonna

"Back in Black" by AC/DC

"Harder to Breathe" by Maroon 5

"Run This Town" (feat. Rihanna and KanYe West) by Jay-Z

"Oops! . . . I Did It Again" by Britney Spears

"Just Dance" by Lady GaGa (feat. Colby O'Donis)

"So What" by P!nk

"Imma Be" by Black Eyed Peas

"Empire State of Mind" (feat. Alicia Keys) by Jay-Z

"Jenny from the Block" by Jennifer Lopez

---

* If you're with your kids at the park, don't just watch from the bench. Get in there and play tag or chase or tee-ball or whatever. See if it doesn't get your heart rate up!

* Wikipedia says you burn 300 calories an hour during sex. Just sayin'.

4. Though I do want you to begin exercising almost every day right away, I also urge you to start carefully and build up strength and endurance so you don't get injured. An injury is a good excuse not to exercise, and I don't want you to have one. So please take it easy and walk before you run, literally. Start with low-impact cardio activities, such as walking and swimming and using the elliptical trainer. When you're ready to try a more strenuous activity, such as running or playing tennis or basketball, start with very short increments of activity and build up your endurance.

5. Be patient. Yes, you're working hard and making some major life changes. But that doesn't mean you'll be exactly where you want to be instantaneously. The longer you've been unhealthy or inactive, the longer it takes. Stick with it. You will get there!

Food

Get ready: This section has some hard-core advice. But I think you can handle it. You're ready. When you're trying to give your diet a swift kick start, it's not the time to mess around.

It's often said that "nothing tastes as good as being thin feels," and while just being thin isn't the goal (you want to be *healthy* and feel and look great), the gist of it is still right. Nothing that you eat can possibly give you as much satisfaction as a fantastic body. A moment on the lips is *not* worth a lifetime on the hips! (Besides, pretty soon you will develop a taste for healthier food, and all the junk will be way less appealing. It really does happen.)

1. Eliminate anything and everything made from white flour from your diet. I'm talking white bread, plain bagels, regular pasta, standard cookies, typical cakes—all those empty carbs. Do it now, all at once, cold turkey. This stuff does absolutely nothing for you, nutritionally speaking. So that means you're just eating meaningless calories. Stop it immediately. I know it sounds harsh. But so often it's easier to have hard-and-fast rules to follow.

2. Eliminate all refined sugar from your diet, too. That's right: no white flour and no white sugar. Of course, refined sugar doesn't always look like white sugar. Anything with high-fructose corn syrup falls into this category as well. So avoid sugary soda, sugary cereals, candy, most cookies, and other sweets.

3. Cut way back on artificial sweeteners, too. Meg Moreta explained to me that when you eat or drink anything artificially sweetened, your metabolism likely slows down. This has been a hot topic in medical research lately, and scientists believe this phenomenon occurs because your body thinks it's getting sugar but

it's not, and so the next time you eat, it could store more calories. What's more, artificially sweetened things can be so sweet that you start craving more and more sweetness. It's a bad cycle you don't want to get trapped in. So don't think fake sweeteners are a diet loophole—they're not. Believe me, I've been hooked on them, too,

---

MD EATS: ✸ *Sample Menu*

Here's what a day of eating looks like for me when I'm cutting out all refined flours and sugars. Looks pretty good, right?

BREAKFAST: Steel-cut oatmeal (a great source of "good" carbs that fill you up and give you energy for the day) mixed with fresh fruit and raw honey as a sweetener. Cinnamon also makes things seem sweet without actually adding sugar. It's a great Jedi mind trick!

SNACK: 1 grapefruit, cut into pieces, mixed with half a Gala apple, also cut into pieces, and tossed with 2 tablespoons fresh mint

LUNCH: Healthy "cobb" salad: baby spinach leaves, ¼ cup chick-peas, chopped egg white from 1 hard-boiled egg, ¼ cup crumbled feta cheese, ½ grilled chicken breast (chopped), tossed with 1 or 2 tablespoons balsamic vinaigrette. Or try the lemon vinaigrette, using the recipe on page 54.

SNACK: Carrots with 1 tablespoon organic natural peanut butter (no sugar added)

DINNER: 1 fillet of salmon, broiled or grilled, with cauliflower puree (see recipe on page 205) and steamed broccoli

and I do still have a Diet Coke or Splenda occasionally when I'm craving something sweet (I figure it's better than a 500-calorie cupcake). But eating them too often can sabotage your best efforts, so it's worth it to cut back, even though it's tough.

4. Eat good food. Have you been wondering what you are allowed to eat since I've told you to cut out so many things? The answer is: Plenty! Vegetables. Fruits. Whole grains. Lean meats. Fish. Beans. Yogurt. Low-fat or skim milk. Nuts. Concentrate on eating whole foods—the closer the food is to its original state, the better it is for you. When you make this way of eating a lifelong habit, staying slim and healthy becomes significantly easier, even if you're not officially "on a diet."

5. Be hyperaware of portion control. If you get used to monitoring your portions carefully, this is a habit that can last you a lifetime. Don't think that the portion a restaurant serves you is the amount you should be eating. Here's what portion sizes should really look like—to give you a sense that portions are actually fairly small:

1 cup of cereal = a baseball

½ cup cooked pasta = a tennis ball

1 ounce cheese = 2 stacked dice

3 ounces meat = a deck of cards

2 tablespoons peanut butter = a golf ball

¼ cup almonds = 12 almonds

MD EATS: ✳ *Cauliflower Puree Recipe*

This is what I make when I'm craving mashed potatoes but want something healthier and with more flavor.

1 medium head cauliflower, roughly chopped
2 garlic cloves
¼ cup chicken stock
¼ cup grated Parmesan cheese
1 tablespoon chopped chives
Salt and pepper to taste

Steam the cauliflower over boiling water until tender. Place it in a food processor or blender.

Lightly toast the garlic cloves in a sauté pan over medium heat for 1 to 2 minutes. Don't let them brown. Remove the garlic from the heat and let cool until you can handle them comfortably. Mince the garlic and add it to the food processor along with the chicken stock, Parmesan cheese, and chopped chives. Pulse until the mixture comes together and reaches a mashed potato–like consistency. Season with salt and pepper to taste.

For foods with nutrition labels, always read the label to find out what constitutes a portion size—and how many portions are in the packages.

6. Commit to drinking at least eight glasses of water per day. (Have I mentioned before how important drinking water is?) Being well hydrated aids weight loss, enables you to exercise more efficiently, and makes your skin look better. If you don't pay attention, it's easy to become dehydrated. When you have

205

the urge to snack, drink a glass of water first. Often when you think you're hungry, you're really just thirsty. And this can make you feel more full between meals.

Fashion

When you're feeling not-so-hot, or heavier than you'd like to be, and you've been feeling that way for a while, getting dressed isn't very much fun. You might not like how you look in things, and because going shopping isn't a pleasure, your wardrobe may be pretty tired and in need of its own kick start!

1. Try on lots of clothes, from your closet and when shopping for new things. You don't need to buy anything—in fact, because you're kick-starting a new healthy regimen, your body may change quite a bit over the coming months, so I wouldn't recommend investing in a new wardrobe at this point. But as you're working toward your goals, trying on clothes can motivate you to stick with it and can start teaching you which styles you like best and work best for you. Try on clothes—things you currently own as well as new clothes—at least every month, so you can gauge your progress, stay motivated, and keep educating yourself about what flatters you.

2. Do a closet purge! Get rid of absolutely everything that makes you feel frumpy. I'm not saying you can't have comfy sweats, but if they make you feel like a total slob, toss 'em. (No, actually, don't toss them—donate them to Goodwill or

a shelter, please. But don't wear them anymore!) Those old sloppy clothes are enabling you to stay in your current slump. You need to get out of your comfort zone!

3. Put together at least one snazzy outfit that looks good and feels great no matter what. We all need at least one of these outfits (and at some point, I want all your outfits to feel that good). This is your go-to outfit. When you have a date night, or a big meeting, wear it with confidence.

4. Promise yourself a splurge on a fabulous outfit when you reach a certain goal, like finishing a 5K race or hitting your goal weight.

Self-Care

Part of kick-starting a healthy lifestyle is taking good care of yourself, in little ways and big ways. If you think about your life and realize you're not doing much of anything that you enjoy, or that you do simply because it feels good (and is good for you), it's time to make some changes.

1. Laugh a lot! Did you know that laughing burns calories? You're doing some major stuff with your diet and your exercise routine right now, and it's hard work. But this doesn't mean you have to be so serious all the time. Have some fun. Watch movies and read books that make you laugh out loud. Write down the hilarious things your kid says, and go back and read them often. This is the best pure comedy around.

(I have more belly laughs doing crazy things with Ben than I ever could have imagined. He is a riot. Recently we acted out a whole conversation based on what we imagined Megan was thinking—since she can't share her thoughts with us just yet. I started it by doing a high-pitched baby-girl voice, and then Ben picked it up, raising his voice to sound like Meggie. We were both cracking up trying to outdo each other with silly, crazy thoughts.) Hang out with the friends who make you laugh. You know who they are—invite them over for dinner (a healthy dinner, of course) and let the funny stories flow.

2. Commit to getting seven to eight hours of sleep every night. Chances are if you've been living a less-than-healthy lifestyle, one of the areas where you've been short-changing yourself is sleep. And sleep is incredibly important if you want to be healthy and look and feel good. Don't underestimate its value! Studies show getting too little sleep can contribute to weight gain and stress; getting enough sleep can contribute to weight loss, improve the appearance of your skin (take a look in the mirror next time you get a good eight hours of shut-eye), and make you more likely to exercise.

3. Treat yourself to a facial (or give yourself one at home—see "Five- or Six-Step DIY Facial" on page 209), and ask the aesthetician for an analysis of your skin and its needs. I know, facials aren't cheap. But we're in kick-start mode, and since your face is the first thing everyone sees and notices about you, it's time to treat it right. A good facial leaves you with clear pores and soft, perfectly moisturized skin. Bonus: It can feel amazing and be totally relaxing.

Make sure you get your money's worth by doing your homework and finding a great facialist (read reviews; get recommendations from friends), and while you're there ask lots of questions about your skin type and what products are best for it. Do you need to be using a richer moisturizer? Exfoliat-

---

MD EXTRA: ✳ *Five- or Six-Step DIY Facial*

This won't give you results quite like you'll get from a professional facial, but it will certainly be good for your skin. And it's easy! When you have thirty minutes or so, give it a try. Do it once a month.

1. Wash your face with a gentle cleanser that's right for your skin type.

2. Exfoliate your skin with a gentle scrub, using a light circular motion and focusing on the areas where your pores might be most clogged.

3. Open your pores by wetting a washcloth with warm (not hot) water and applying it to your face for ten to fifteen seconds. Repeat three times.

4. Apply a facial mask appropriate for your skin type—a hydrating mask for dry skin, or a clay-based mask for oily skin. Follow the directions for the product you choose.

5. If desired, apply a toner that's right for your skin type.

6. Apply a moisturizer, again choosing one that's right for your skin type—rich and hydrating for dry skin; lighter and maybe oil-free for oily skin.

---

ing more often? Applying a vitamin C serum? Learn what will help you glow. Tip: You don't need to buy the expensive products sold at the spa—ask for more general recommendations and shop around for lower-priced versions.

4. Go to the dentist. Does this seem like a weird suggestion? Well, going to the dentist might not be fun, but one of the most important parts of how you look is your smile. When was the last time you went to the dentist for a cleaning? Don't you remember how great your teeth feel afterward? (Plus, regular dentist appointments—along with regular brushing and flossing—are key to good oral health. It's better to go to the dentist now than to have a root canal and ten cavities later.) If it's been longer than you can remember, book an appointment today. It's not a bad idea to get those whitening strips while you're at it. There's no need to go all crazy for the "Chiclets" look, but whiter teeth could give you the confidence to smile brightly when meeting someone for the first time.

5. You're doing all this hard work, so learn how to show off your new body. For one thing, stand up straight. (See, Mom, I was listening.) Have you thought about your posture lately? I bet if you straightened your spine right now you'd be at least an inch taller. How you stand and how you hold yourself physically can make a huge difference to how you look. Not only are you taller, you're thinner, too! Ask any professional dancer (or just take my word for it, since I know a few) and she'll agree. Use those stomach muscles to hold you up; mentally picture yourself stacking one vertebra on top of the other. If you do that all the way up, your shoulders should fall a little

bit back, which makes your chest stick out a little, and that's a good thing. It's hard to change your posture overnight, so pick a certain time of day, or a certain trigger, something that reminds you to correct your posture, and see if you can make a habit of standing up straight, too.

Romance

I suspect that some of you who've let many months or years pass without taking good care of yourself may also have let many months or years pass without taking good care of your relationship. And by "taking good care of your relationship" I don't mean folding your husband's laundry or picking up his dry cleaning (though that's nice of you, and I hope he returns the favor!). I mean spending quality time together, really talking, and being reminded often why you love each other. Here are some nice—and healthy—ways to reconnect:

1. Exercise together. When you have kids, I know this isn't always easy—for many of your workouts, he's probably on kid duty. Still, as they say, the couple that plays together stays together. You can inspire each other, do things you both think are fun, and encourage each other to stick with your respective fitness routines. So have a friend, relative, or sitter stay with your kid(s) occasionally, and turn a workout into a date. Dave and I take the kids out for hikes, and our gym has a kids' club, so we all go together to the gym sometimes. Dave also taught me to play racquetball. It was so much fun, and one of the hardest workouts ever because I was so

competitive. I wanted to win! So I was running all over the court, killing myself to keep up with Dave. We had fun, and good stories to laugh about later, mostly at my expense.

2. Cook dinner together. (And then eat it together!) When you make dinner at home instead of going out or picking up take-out, the chances that you'll eat healthful foods are much better because you control every ingredient. After the kids have gone to bed, turn on some (quiet) music, light a few candles, and whip up a healthy feast. It doesn't have to be complicated—simple, straightforward foods are often the healthiest, actually. One of the most fun Valentine's Days Dave planned for me was one where we spent the evening in a fancy kitchen learning how to make a gourmet meal with a few other couples, and then we sat down to enjoy the amazing meal we had helped prepare. Don't wait for V-Day to make dinner with your hubby.

3. While you're eating the healthy dinner you prepared together, really focus on each other. One way to do this is to write out some questions in advance that you want to ask. They can be deep questions (What's your biggest dream for the future? What are your goals for our family?) or sexy questions (What are your fantasies? What was your favorite thing about the first night we slept together?) or "Proust Questionnaire" questions (Where would you live if you could live anywhere? When and where were you happiest?) Google "Proust Questionnaire" to find more or ask whatever kind of questions you want. Over a candlelit meal, ask the questions and let the intimacy flow from there.

Mommy Maintenance

Everyone talks about how hard it is to lose weight and get fit, but sometimes it's harder to *stay* in good shape once you get there. You have adrenaline flowing while you're trying to reach your goals, and the excitement is less obvious when the aim is to maintain status quo. Maybe that's why, unfortunately, we all know people who are constantly yo-yo dieting, and even on *The Biggest Loser* we sometimes see former contestants gaining weight back.

To make maintenance work for you, you've got to change your way of thinking about it. Maintaining your health and fitness and working out and being in great shape—none of that is boring! It's awesome. Think about how great you feel, and how fantastic you look, and all the things you can do with your body, whether you want to keep up with your baby as she starts walking or, hey, run a marathon! Whatever you want to do, you can do it.

Maintaining "Mommy Diet" shape isn't just about eating right and exercising, of course. Taking care of *you* needs to be a regular and ongoing part of your life. You need to keep getting sleep, pampering yourself, and wearing cute outfits. You do not need to give up and resign yourself to a life of mom jeans, baggy sweatshirts, and sensible shoes. Be a hot mom!

Fitness

When I was finally back in shape after having Megan, I didn't stop pushing myself. If anything, I was more excited than ever about my workouts. They felt so good, and I could work harder and accomplish more. One day when Megan was about ten months old, I went to *The Biggest Loser* campus to work out at the BL gym. I'm always so inspired working out on campus. Something about the energy there just gets me moving. So I decided to run sprints on the treadmill, and it felt amazing. And then some of the contestants from season nine and I decided to spin together. (Yes, after my treadmill sprints. I really wanted to. I promise, after a while, working out feels that good!) Drea, Stephanie, Sherry, Sunshine, Ashley, Sam, and I were all there, spinning together. They were only five weeks into the show, and I was so impressed by how hard they worked. We pulled the bikes into a circle and motivated one another, and we bonded over the music (the mix we used that day is on page 218). I was reminded again how amazing it feels to be in shape, to push your body to work hard, and to enjoy all the things that are good for you.

1. Mix things up. If you do the same workout—say, thirty minutes on the treadmill at exactly the same speed and incline every

time—it's going to be really tough to stick with it because it's boring. You will start to dread it. And your body will get used to it, so the workout will be less and less effective at challenging muscles and burning calories. If you're in a rut, get out of it! Check out different cardio machines at the gym. Walk or run a more interesting route (look for trails, or hills, or a sandy beach). Go to a new class. I love trying different types of workouts. My friend Denise Richards and I have tried a couple different classes together. One class we tried, at Bar Method, totally kicked my butt. Literally: My behind was in pain afterward. It's a super-intense workout, and yet you don't move much at all. It was such a good lesson in how controlling your own muscles and resistance work can be exhausting and very effective. I know I'm not describing it well, but trust me, if you ever get the chance . . . try it. Be prepared to feel sore in muscles you didn't know you had. That's the beauty of a different workout.

2. Have fun. The more you like the things you do for exercise, the more likely you are to do them. Simple, yes, but so many people forget that a workout can be—gasp—enjoyable! One of the reasons I go to spin class so often is because I love it. I have fun there. Yes, it challenges me and pushes me and makes me sweat. But it's a great time, too. It's always different, the music pumps me up, and the camaraderie with the others in the class is cool—you're all in it together. Maybe spin will be a favorite of yours. Maybe you love to run. Or play tennis. Or do yoga. Or snowshoe. Or play soccer. Or do kickboxing. Or do a striptease-style dance class. (Hey, whatever gets you moving!) Or all of the above. If you like it, do it—often.

3. Be consistent. Ideally you'll be working out at least three days a week, and preferably more than that. But you're a busy mom, so finding time for that isn't easy. You need to make time. What I do is tell myself I will work out every day that I can. There will always be days when it's impossible to squeeze in a workout. But by committing to work out every single day when I can, I end up getting in a healthy number of workouts every week. It's not easy, I know. It takes focus and drive, and you're the only one who can make it happen. (As I said at the beginning of this book, you have to want it!) But you can do it, and it's so worth it.

4. Don't set impossible workout goals—be realistic about your time and attention span. Dave has a routine that lasts about forty minutes at the gym. He told me it's long enough to get in a good workout but short enough that he'll actually go and do it. If you're forcing yourself to do superlong workouts that you don't enjoy, or don't have time for, you'll end up just making excuses not to go, and you won't get any workout in. Limit your time at the gym enough that you'll actually go do it, and then be sure to use the time wisely while you're there.

5. Mix up the intensity. As you're trying out new workouts, you'll see that not all classes are created equal. If you've been pushing yourself to get into good shape, by the time you hit maintenance mode, you're pretty athletic, which means a lot of workouts people think are "tough". . . well . . . aren't. So don't be surprised if you sign up for a class and leave feeling like you didn't get a tough workout. Don't be disappointed—it's impor-

tant that you learn to push yourself, but it's also good to not go full speed *all the time*. One night, I took a spin class with a new teacher. She played more mellow music than my regular instructor and didn't yell at me to up the intensity. As a result, I had a so-so workout and I talked to my trainer about it. She said it's not always necessary to go "balls to the wall" and that sometimes it's good to let your body get a mellower workout in. I'm a type A person, and I'm sure the expression on my face was saying, "Um, what? That doesn't compute." But after we talked it through for a while, I realized she's right. It's good to work out at different levels, and good to go for a nice hike instead of an intense run sometimes. That being said, I still generally prefer dripping with sweat after spending an hour in the gym. It makes me feel satisfied. But I try to take my trainer's advice and break it up once in a while.

6. Wear workout clothes that are both comfortable and confidence boosting. Volleyball star and model Gabrielle Reece has been a guest on *The Biggest Loser* several times, and during Season 9 she talked to the contestants about the importance of workout clothes that fit well and look great. She's right. If you're wearing, say, an oversized, ratty T-shirt and unflattering shorts, you aren't going to want to work out where someone might see you. Don't let that become an excuse for skipping exercise. I am always much happier at the gym or on a hike when I think I'm in a good workout outfit. It shouldn't be crazy stylish or cutesy or anything, just appropriate—something that adds to your confidence instead of detracting from it. Of course, it has to move well with you and be functional,

MD TUNES: ❋ *Fun Spin Playlist*

This is the mix we listened to when I did the spin class with the contestants from Season 9 of *The Biggest Loser*. Love it!

"Use Somebody" by Kings of Leon (perfect warm-up song)

"Put On" by Young Jeezy feat. KanYe West (a good "out of the saddle" fast trot, this gets your blood pumping)

"No One" by Alicia Keys (our first climb up the hill)

"Hard to Handle" (Live) by The Black Crowes (racing down the hill)

"Mr. E's Beautiful Blues" by Eels (another good beat to trot to)

"Bring Me to Life" by Evanescence (a good upbeat trot, this song gives you a chance to get your heart rate back down a bit)

"This Ain't a Scene, It's an Arms Race" by Fall Out Boy (we used the chorus to come in and out of the saddle)

"Billie Jean" by Michael Jackson (a great song for losing yourself in the workout)

"So What" by P!nk (a good song to help you fight through the exhaustion)

"Halo" by Beyoncé (this played for the BIG hill in our ride: stay in the saddle and turn up the tension!)

"Mr. Brightside" by The Killers (reduce the tension only a little. . . you're still on the hill)

"In the End" by Linkin Park (now race back down the hill)

"I'm Yours" by Jason Mraz (a fun way to finish up a tough workout—you can't help but be happy with this tune)

too—I like outfits that make me feel like an athlete! When I first started working out again after Megan was born, I favored capris that widen at the bottom and longer shirts to ensure that my belly wasn't showing when I lifted my arms. I think I wore maternity tanks at the gym for the six months after Megan was born. I have one that says "mother of 2" on it, and it was my defense mechanism. It was long and slightly loose, and hell, it made me feel comfortable and confident, so whatever works! Loose yoga pants were a favorite then, too. But now that I feel more confident about my figure (I had to wear a bikini on *Days* just recently; after that, nothing scares me!) I wear more fitted stretch pants or running pants. I find it does help for running and spinning not to have a lot of extra fabric around the ankle. Nike and Lululemon are two of my favorite brands of athletic clothing. Both make lots of pieces that are cute, fitted, and athletic without seeming too . . . anything. Once you have a sense of your best workout outfits, stock up on a few so you can't use the "it's in the laundry" excuse, either.

Food

Adopting a healthy diet while you're trying to get back in great shape and then going right back to unhealthy habits doesn't work. Does. Not. Work.

In order to keep feeling and looking fabulous, those good eating habits need to be yours for a lifetime. Does that mean you have to be totally perfect all the time and never even look at another cupcake for the rest of your life? No! It's okay to indulge a little . . . occasionally. As Meg Moreta says, if you're really good 90 percent of the time, you have a little leeway with the other 10 percent. But don't live for that 10 percent— enjoy being a healthy eater. Here are some tips to help you stick with it all the time. Okay, almost all the time!

1. Keep a food journal. Ugh, I know, this is no fun and it sounds like a chore. I'll be honest: It *is* a chore. (Plus, sometimes it would be nice to eat a cookie and not have to write about it later.) But it helps you to keep track of what you're eating, at every meal and over the course of a day, a week, a month. Then you'll know if there are certain times of day when you struggle, and you'll know, if you had a splurge-heavy day, that you need to be careful for the next few days. Plus, it forces you to acknowledge every single thing you eat. Even if it's just a bite or a spoonful of something, write it down. No cheating! (Come on, do not lie in your own food journal—that's just counterproductive.) Meg told me that keeping a food journal is one of the best predictors of weight loss and weight maintenance success. I strongly suggest doing it, even if you don't feel like it.

2. Be aware of calories, and be honest with yourself about how many you're consuming. Sure, it's fine to treat yourself once in a while. But be aware of what you're doing, and know the calorie count and sugar content. Don't pretend it's not that bad, or ignore the reality of what you're consuming. A lot of people who gain weight do so unknowingly. Working at *The Biggest Loser* has taught me a lot about caloric intake. I know

how many calories are in so many tasty, tempting treats now, and I know that it does no good to fool yourself about what you're eating. Read labels and know what portion sizes are, too. There's a "healthy" granola out there with 200 calories and 10 grams of fat per serving. But a serving size is ¼ cup! How many people pour only ¼ cup of cereal in the morning, unless they are conscious of calories? A quarter cup is tiny! So check portion sizes as well as calorie counts. Oh yeah, and if there's

MD EATS: ☀ *Calorie Counts*

Here are some calorie counts to keep in mind next time you're thinking of eating something you know is a splurge but want to pretend isn't.

CUPCAKE: 500 to 800 calories

DOUGHNUT: 220 to 450 calories

BAGEL: 200 to 500 calories (that's *without* cream cheese)

CAESAR SALAD: 700 calories or more

FAST-FOOD BURGER: 250 to 500 calories and up

LARGE (*not* **"supersized"**) **FAST-FOOD FRENCH FRIES:** 500 calories

FRIED CHICKEN (one serving): 900 calories

PINT OF BEN & JERRY'S CHUBBY HUBBY ICE CREAM: 1,320 calories (If you can't stop after just one bite, don't do it!)

Look for more calorie counts at alisonsweeney.com.

no label, don't think it's calorie-free! Be realistic about your assessment—a giant chocolate-chip cookie from the bakery has more than 100 calories, people. A lot more.

3. Be smart when you eat out. I have to eat out a lot—on-set meals are basically like restaurants. You'd think the television industry could figure out how to offer only healthy foods so it's easier to stay in shape, but nope! There's a sea of creamy sauces and fat-laden dressings to navigate, not to mention all the bagels and bread and pasta and sweets. When faced with all these choices, don't forget everything you know about healthy eating. Because what you eat when you're out has just as much of an impact on your body as what you eat at home. The rules don't change! Here are some guidelines for navigating menus when eating out:

* *Cheesy, creamy,* and *fried* are adjectives to avoid.

* Salads are great, but not if they're loaded with fatty dressing, bacon bits, cheese, and other unhealthy add-ons. Read the ingredients carefully, and if it's a heavy dressing, ask them to replace it with a light vinaigrette (or get the dressing on the side, and use it sparingly). And if you order a salad with chicken, be sure to ask for grilled or broiled chicken (often the chicken is fried). It's your right as a customer to ask for a healthier version of the salad. And perhaps you'll encourage the chef to offer smarter options.

* Skip the bread basket. Just skip it. I mentioned this earlier—it's such a simple thing to do. Ask your

server not to bring it so you're never even tempted. Why fill up on empty calories before your meal arrives?

* Practice portion control. If you're in a place that you know has huge portions, plan to take home half of your meal in a doggy bag. And remember that it's perfectly okay to order an appetizer as an entrée. The portions are smaller—closer to what you actually should be having as an entrée portion! Or split the entrée with your hubby. Dave and I often split a meal instead of ordering our own entrées. Stay away from the kids' menu if you think that's a good place to go for smaller portions. Yes, they might be smaller, but the food generally isn't healthy. We never order for Ben from a kids' menu. We want him to experience a range of flavors and textures, and not get used to mac-and-cheese and hot dogs.

* Intentionally order foods that you know are healthy. You know this stuff! Look for things like grilled chicken and fish and vegetables. Steer clear of heavy pasta dishes, and that double cheeseburger with fries, and the molten chocolate cake with ice cream. (If you want to try something decadent, share it, just have a bite or two, and remember that those little bites do contain fat and calories!)

MD EATS: ✳ *Grown-Up Popsicles*

When you just want a taste of something sweet—and don't want to blow your calorie budget—try a homemade popsicle. Ben received a popsicle maker for his birthday, and we have fun making juice-based treats for him, so I thought, *Why not make them for grownups, too?* You can find very affordable 3- or 4-ounce BPA-free popsicle molds on Amazon.com or at kitchen supply stores. Or you can make little "pops" in an ice cube tray. We have 4-ounce popsicle molds, and the popsicles I make each have 40 calories or less. Play around with different juices, fruits, and herbs and come up with your own delicious concoctions. Here are two of my favorites:

POMEGRANATE PUNCH POPSICLES
Makes two 4-ounce pops

Pour ½ cup *diet* lemon-lime soda (such as Sprite or 7Up) into a liquid measuring cup with a pour spout. Let it sit at room temperature for 5 minutes to go somewhat flat. (This is an important step. If you get antsy and skip it, your pop will be filled with air bubbles and overflow when frozen.) Stir ½ cup pomegranate juice (such as POM) into the soda. Pour the mixture into the popsicle forms and follow the manufacturer's instructions for freezing.

→

4. When you have a major craving, give in to it. But just a little. Instead of a giant muffin, have a mini muffin. Rather than a huge cupcake with an enormous swirl of icing, try a mini cupcake. My best friend gave me an ice cream maker for my birthday last year, which may seem like a cruel gift, given that she knows I'm trying to be healthy, but she understands

LEMON POPSICLES WITH MINT AND APPLE

Makes two 4-ounce pops

Combine ½ cup freshly squeezed lemon juice with ½ cup water in a liquid measuring cup with a pour spout. Sweeten with a teaspoon of raw sugar (15 calories per teaspoon), ½ teaspoon of Agave nectar (about 10 calories per ½ teaspoon), or your favorite calorie-free sweetener. (This should taste like very intense lemonade.) Chiffonade (which means cut into long, thin strips) 4 or 5 mint leaves (or try basil leaves for a sophisticated twist) and mix them into the lemonade. Pour the lemonade into popsicle forms, add one or two very thin apple slices to each form, and follow the manufacturer's instructions for freezing.

that I love experimenting and making different flavors, and that I can make some and have just one bite, because it's the real deal. And I'd rather do that than have a whole portion of sugar-free ice cream (which doesn't even taste that good, and isn't really good for you either with all that artificial crap in it). When you really, really want something, don't eat ten other things in an attempt to make the craving go away. You'll end up eating lots of calories and other stuff you don't need, and you won't be satisfied.

5. If there's something you can't resist, don't have it in the house! This is pretty simple. If the temptation isn't physically there, you can't give in to it. Why stock your freezer full of ice cream and keep your cookie jar full if you know you'll polish off way too much in

one sitting? You can use other tricks to avoid junk, too. For example, I love to bake with Ben, and he loves to lick the beater! When we make cookies, I put nuts or raisins in them because I don't like nuts or raisins in my cookies. So after the cookies are baked, I don't worry about eating them, because I know I won't.

6. If you overindulge once (or more), do not give up on the whole day or week. Believe me, I know how it goes: One bite leads to another, and another, and another, and suddenly I've cheated three times and I feel like the whole day is ruined before dinner. Instead of throwing the whole day away, pick yourself up and say, *Okay, I have to make up for this on the other end*. Eat something light for dinner, and for breakfast and lunch the next day, and be sure to have a good workout. I get it, and it's hard, but you can stick with it. One slipup is not the end of the world—and definitely not the end of a healthy diet!

Fashion

There's no denying that when you love how you look in an outfit—no matter what you're wearing—your confidence and overall mood get a boost (even if just a small one). On the other hand, when you don't like what you're wearing on a given day, chances are you don't feel quite as perky.

Whether you're a crazed stay-at-home mom or you have to rush, rush, rush to get ready to go to work in the morning, it makes sense to put some thought into getting dressed. Because when you feel better about yourself, it's that much easier to be good to those around you. Don't get frustrated or give up because you think fashion doesn't come naturally to you. As my stylist, Liza, always reminds me, everyone who dresses well needs to work at it. She points out that Sarah Jessica Parker, one of the world's most popular style icons, had five-hour fittings and try-on sessions every week while filming *Sex and the City*. She was working with one of the best stylists in the country, Patricia Field, and it still took that long! So don't expect that you will look perfectly chic without putting in the effort. Here are some tips for becoming your own style icon:

1. Be in good shape. Stay in good shape. The truth is that clothes will look and feel better on you when your body is in healthy shape. (And then seeing how great you look in your clothes can help motivate you to stick with healthy eating and exercise. It's a positive cycle that you can perpetuate forever!)

2. Try on. Try on. Try on. Get in the habit of trying clothes on, at the store and at home. Never buy something you haven't tried on—it might look good on the hanger, but that doesn't mean it will look good on you. And don't just pull one thing off the rack and give up if it doesn't fit. It takes some hunting to find things that fit me off the rack, though lately (thanks to designers making petite lines for height-challenged people like me) I've been having a little more luck. Try on the clothes you already own, too, honestly assessing how they look on you. I'm not saying you should ditch something that doesn't fit two weeks after you have a baby. But when you're back in shape, check yourself out from head to toe in any outfit you plan to

wear. Don't like how it looks? Don't wear it. Try on the stuff you don't wear very often, too—you might find a surprisingly fabulous new look.

3. Learn what looks good on you, and don't try to force a look that doesn't work (even if it's totally in right now and looks phenomenal on your best friend). I have a really long waist and short legs, so not all pant and skirt lengths look good on me. Capris and midcalf-length skirts cut me off and make me look ridiculous. It's frustrating, too, because often, there are supercute flowy skirts that are pretty and fun, but not right for me.

4. Take care of your clothes. Stained, torn, or pilled clothes look messy and unkempt. A coat with buttons missing isn't quite as polished as it could be. Do a quick scan of your clothes before you put them away, and if there's anything that needs repairing or cleaning, do it right away. I can't tell you how many times I've put a shirt back in my closet because it has a stain on it, only to pull it out another day for a repeat of that moment. It's like putting an empty milk carton back in the fridge. Why bother? Decide what to do with it: Have it cleaned? Donate it? Do it right away, while you're in the moment!

5. Get to know a good tailor. Unless you can afford custom couture for everyday—can anyone afford that?—you'll be buying clothes off the rack. And while I really don't suggest buying anything that doesn't look great on you, there are probably pieces in your closet that you love that would look much better with just a little tweak or two, maybe a nip in at the

waist or a shortening of the sleeve. Oh, and jeans and pants: Why are they almost all cut to fit six-foot-tall supermodels? Unless they are from a designer who does a great petites line, I usually need to have mine shortened a lot. Ask your tailor to keep the original hem on jeans—it looks so much cooler. When men buy pants or a new suit, they are much more likely than women to get them tailored to fit. But women's bodies are so much more unique and complicated—we should all be using tailors more often to make clothes fit us better. It's cheaper than going out and buying something new!

6. Clean out your closet! It sounds counterintuitive, but it's true: When you have fewer clothes in your closet, it will feel like you have more that you actually want to wear. The key is editing your wardrobe often, and removing those things you've been hanging on to for years that you never end up wearing. Those are getting in the way of the stuff that looks good on you, and distracting you from your great outfits. My rule? If I haven't worn it for more than a year (unless it's a very-special-occasion piece), it goes. Trust me, this is a huge time-saver. Just get rid of the clothes you don't love and you'll have a closet full of viable options. It's okay if there's not much left in there, because as long as you love what you have, you'll always look and feel good. And again, don't throw your castoffs into the trash—give them to a friend, donate them to a shelter or Goodwill, or make a little money by selling them at a consignment shop. Or if they're really good pieces, but just not right for you anymore, plan a fun clothing swap night with your girlfriends. If you have a few friends with similar shoe or dress sizes, lay out all the stuff

you don't want, have them bring their stuff, and start trading! It's fun—have some wine and enjoy the "shopping!"

Self-Care

One of the biggest lessons I hope you take away from this book is that it's a good thing to take care of yourself. That means more than working out and eating well (though those things are part of the equation for sure). I'm talking about all the little things that help you look and feel fantastic: taking care of your skin and hair, putting on makeup, getting a pedicure, getting a massage, getting a facial, reading, watching a chick flick . . . whatever works for you. When you become a mom, it's a whole lot harder to make time for things like this. (Yup, it's a whole lot harder to make time for pretty much everything.) But it's important, for you and your whole family. When you feel good, you will have the capacity and energy to be a better mom.

1. Book self-care into your schedule. Christie suggests picking one day per week and promising yourself that you will treat yourself to some form of pampering on that day, every week, without fail. (She does it on Thursdays. Usually Sundays are my day.) It can be anything from picking up your favorite celebrity magazine and reading it over a cup of tea to something more involved, like getting a haircut and highlights. Whether you spend five minutes or, hello, five hours at the spa (aaah . . . yes, I know this won't happen very often!), make this as much a part of your routine as grocery shopping and doctor's appointments. Enjoy

the little things, too. For example, I *love* going to the grocery store. Seriously. It's such a relaxing thing for me to stroll up and down the aisles picking out good produce and deciding what to make for dinner that week. Wow, when I wrote that I realized it's even geekier than I thought. But it's true!

2. Get enough sleep. This is one of the most important things you can do for your health, for your looks (seriously—getting enough sleep is key for good skin), and for your psyche. I've already mentioned a few times how important it is to try to get eight hours. But if that's not possible, and believe me, I hear *that,* maybe fit in a catnap in the afternoon. Set your alarm and shut your eyes! You will probably really feel refreshed from the self-imposed time-out. And try to hit the sack a little earlier at night. You've got a wonderful little alarm clock now, and if she's awake for the day at 6 a.m., so are you. (I won't even mention the 2 a.m. and 4 a.m. wake-ups here—if you're already a mom, you know all about those, and if you're expecting your first, well, you'll find out!)

Romance

No matter how busy you get with your kids, no matter what else life throws at you, always prioritize your relationship. (In most cases, you wouldn't have kids if it weren't for your relationship!)

1. Have I mentioned before how important communication is? Good. It's worth bringing up again. Talk to each other, all the

time. Say what's on your mind, whether it seems monumentally important or trivial.

2. Plan for plenty of alone time. Time slips away quickly. You might wake up and realize that a month or two or six have flown by, and you can't remember the last time you and your husband went on a date. Or even had an hour alone together. Do your best to ensure that doesn't happen. A regular date night (every week or every other week) is *not* too much to ask!

3. Be proactive. When you realize that you both are in a rut, or starting to fall into a rut . . . make a change! Don't let more time slip away. Do something surprising and romantic. *You* plan the date. Or leave a note in his car, or surprise him with a picnic, or just whisper sweet nothings in his ear as you watch TV tonight. Want to have sex? Just go for it. Guys are not really big on reading subtlety, as you've no doubt figured out by now. Make your overtures loud and clear, and embrace their surprised and pleased reactions. (You don't need me to get graphic here, do you? If you need more suggestions, tune in to *Days of Our Lives*.)

4. Shake things up. "Maintenance" (in fitness, nutrition, *and* romance) is not just about doing the same thing day in and day out. It has to be a roller coaster. That's part of the fun. Maintaining your romantic relationship with your husband is definitely going to be filled with highs and lows. Just don't let the lows last too long, and always enjoy the ride.

MD EXTRA: ❋ *A Few Parting Thoughts*

Recently I took a Zen spin class: The room was lit with candles, and a Zen master shared wisdom with us while we worked out. That might sound hokey, but it was inspiring. He reminded us how important it is to emit positive energy, because, he said, the energy that we give off comes back to us. If you sit around feeling sorry for yourself, the things you want just aren't going to come to you. However, if you think you *can* do something, you *will* be able to do it. If you believe in yourself, others will believe in you.

Even when there's not a Zen master guiding me through my workout, spin class is where a lot of my clearest thinking happens. Theres's something about all that physical exertion that enables me to cut through the bull and focus. And that's when I think hard about what motivates me. In this book I've shared plenty of tips for getting healthy and fit; as you follow them, please don't forget to spend time considering *why* you're doing all this. Your reasons should be personal and deeply felt. If your motivation or inspiration is weak, your results will be, too. Don't let that happen. As you take the journey toward looking and feeling great, make sure you know what's driving you, and that you are committed to *you*.

These are important things to remember as you review all the information in this book and work to get in (and stay in) great shape before and during your pregnancy, and when you are a mom. As long as you have the right attitude, you have everything you need. You just need to *do it*. As I've said before, there are no shortcuts, no secret buttons to press, and no magic tricks—and no one can do it for you. There's no way around sweating and eating right and taking care of yourself. Hard work is the only way to do it right.

Please believe that you can do this. I believe in you, too.

Acknowledgments

I have always loved to read. When I was a kid, my dad would catch me reading in my closet in the middle of the night— it was the perfect hideout because my parents couldn't see the light on. To have a book with my name on it, to share my thoughts, and to think that maybe someone, somewhere, is reading it late into the night (as I still do) is an amazing thrill for me.

One thing I didn't think about all those years ago, Laura Ingalls Wilder book in hand, was just how many people go into the making of one book—how many people help, guide, support, and edit the author toward the final product. This book is certainly no different.

I have to start by thanking my coauthor, Christie Matheson. I loved our long conference calls, which occasionally took place as one of us was feeding a baby or soothing tears— multitasking as only a mom can. We have a lot in common, and also some differences, too, which I think helped us to provide readers with broader and more useful information.

My mom, Polly, set an excellent example right from the beginning of what it's like to be a great working mom. She taught me to love what I do and to work hard always to be the best I can be in everything I pursue.

I am so proud to have surrounded myself with strong, dynamic women who believe in me and have been such fantastic supporters: Barbara Rubin, Hayley Lozitsky, and Stephanie, Lauren, Melissa, Corina, Deidre, and Liza.

This is a book about living a healthy lifestyle, so of course I have to thank Mark Koops and everyone in *The Biggest Loser* family. I've learned so much being a part of such a positive, inspiring, and educational show.

Tricia Boczkowski has been an excellent guide and supporter at Gallery Books, and I'm happy to work with the amazing team there.

Jane Dystel, my literary agent, has been fantastic, and I am so grateful to her for introducing me to Christie. Thank you to Michael Camacho, Max Stubblefield, Ennis Kamcili, Jacob Fenton, and everyone on my team at UTA. They have been essential in pushing me to pursue my professional goals and helping me see them through.

I have several people who cross over between my personal and professional lives, none more vital than my dad, Stender. I couldn't have done any of this without him. He's guided me, encouraged me, and never been afraid to reprimand me when I needed it. And he's always been the first person to believe in me, and ask only "How can I help?"

For more than fifteen years (yikes) Carrie Simons has been my best friend and co-conspirator, and now she could claim about nine different job titles in my professional life, if she wanted. I'm so blessed to have her on my side.

My husband, Dave, and I have been married for more than ten years now, and we keep growing closer and stronger together. He's an amazing partner, and I love how he challenges me and supports me when I need it, and also provides me with a total escape from Hollywood when I need that. We have two beautiful children, Ben and Megan. Dave, Ben, and Megan are the three most important people in my life. My heart is so full of love for them, and I am beyond grateful for each of them. (And I'm lucky that Dave can sleep with my book-light on late into the night.)